Nicola M. Hall trained in medicine at S̲and subsequently worked in a wide varimore interested in the field of alternativin Reflexology with Mrs Doreen Bayly (a pupil of the pioneer Eunice Ingham) in 1977, assisting her with her training courses at the Bayly School of Reflexology until Mrs Bayly died in 1979. Nicola Hall then took over as Director of the School in 1980. She is also Chairman of the British Reflexology Association. She lives in Worcestershire.

St. Mary's Hospital Medical School.
ry of jobs, becoming more and
medicine. She began her training

Reflexology – A Way to Better Health

Foot and hand massage for relaxation and treating many ailments

Nicola M. Hall

Illustrated by Jim Howden

Pan Original
Pan Books London, Sydney and Auckland

First published 1988 by Pan Books Ltd,
Cavaye Place, London SW10 9PG

9 8 7 6 5 4 3 2

© Nicola M. Hall 1988

Illustrations © Nicola M. Hall 1988

ISBN 0 330 30208 6

Printed and bound in Great Britain by Richard Clay Ltd.

Acknowledgements

Kirlian Photography between pages 96–97 thanks to Graham Wilson of The London Natural Health Clinic, Arnica House, 170 Campden Hill Road, London W8 7AS.

Acupressure points chart on pages 169–70 is based on information in *Do-It-Yourself Shiatsu* by Wataru Ohashi (Mandala Books).

The meridians in the foot chart on page 171 are based on information in a chart produced by Jan van Baarle, Amsterdam, The Netherlands.

Contents

		page
	Introduction	9
1	Reflexology — What is it About?	11
2	The Reflex Areas of the Feet and the Hands	27
3	How Reflexology Treatment is Given — The Massage Technique	103
4	Foot and Hand Care	113
5	How the Treatment works	115
6	The Treatment Session	121
7	The Treatment of Different Disorders	123
8	Examples of Treatment	157
9	Other Treatments Involving the Feet and the Hands	167
10	Reflexology Around the World	177
	Useful Addresses	181
	Index	183

Introduction

The curative effects of massage have been known for many years and the popularity of this type of treatment has been revived more recently with the increased awareness and acceptance of the 'alternative' or 'complementary' therapies.

Reflexology is a particular form of massage which involves working with the thumbs and in some instances the fingers on reflex areas which are found in the feet and the hands. By massaging these reflex points, it is possible to treat the different areas of the body since every part of the feet and the hands corresponds to a specific part of the body. In a Reflexology treatment session, the whole of both feet or both hands will be massaged to treat the whole body. It is more common for Reflexology to be applied by a practitioner to the feet, though the hands are more easily worked on for self-treatment. It is a method which is used to treat many ailments and most people will feel benefit afterwards.

In addition to its use as a treatment of ill-health, Reflexology can be used to maintain good health, as a prevention of illness. Through the accurate diagnosis obtained from massaging the reflex areas of the feet or the hands, health problems can be detected early on and treatment given to prevent serious symptoms from developing. Another great benefit of the treatment is its use as a means of relaxation. So many people nowadays suffer from stress, tension and the inability to relax, all of which can lead to ill-health. A Reflexology treatment session is an easy and extremely pleasant way of helping the body to relax.

Probably one of the biggest disadvantages of Reflexology is its simplicity. People will inevitably be sceptical about the fact that by massaging the feet or the hands, all sorts of different problems can be alleviated but do not be put off by its simplicity.

To a certain extent, Reflexology is a therapy which you can try on yourself but for best results it is sensible to visit a qualified practitioner who will be an expert on the correct application. In this way you will feel the wonderful effects of the treatment, as described in this book. You will also soon become aware of the great importance of the feet and the hands not only for their normal daily tasks but also as a reflection of the body and its state of health.

1 Reflexology – What is it About?

Reflexology is the name given to the form of treatment which involves giving massage in a certain manner to all of the areas of the feet. In the feet there are reflex areas which relate to all the parts of the body, and these reflex areas are found on the soles, the top, and the sides of the feet. In fact, the feet as a whole correspond to the whole of the body in a manner which will be described later. By massaging the various areas, a diagnosis of the parts of the body which are out of balance, and therefore not working efficiently, can be made and treatment given to correct these imbalances and thus return the body to good working order. In addition to the reflex areas found in the feet, similar reflex areas exist in the hands, again corresponding to the whole of the body. The hands can be used for treatment also, though the feet are usually preferred by the practitioner since they are normally more responsive. The feet offer a larger area to be treated and since they are generally protected by shoes and socks they present a more sensitive area for the treatment than the hands. The hands are used when it is not possible to work on the feet and they do lend themselves more readily as the area to be worked on in self-treatment. Although the hands may not be as sensitive as the feet initially, they will become more sensitive to the method when worked on with Reflexology massage.

How the Therapy Developed

In order to understand how the reflex areas are arranged in the feet and hands and how these were determined, it is helpful to look at the history of the method.

Many thousands of years ago in China, the ancient Chinese practised various forms of medicine quite different from those of the Western world. The most famous of these must be acupuncture, which involves inserting needles into certain areas of the body known as acupuncture points. These points are situated on lines known as meridian lines which are 'energy' lines distributed throughout the body and, by placing a needle at a certain point, energy within a meridian can be redistributed which will result in a correction of an ailment associated with this meridian. Often a needle is inserted in an area quite distant from the actual part of the body requiring treatment but is effective since it is linked to that part of the body by the meridian line. Reflexology is based on similar ideas to acupuncture in that there are energy lines linking the feet and the hands to the various body parts and the whole body can be treated by working on the reflex areas in the feet and hands. The energy lines of Reflexology are not, however, the same as the acupuncture meridian lines but the system obviously has its origins in these ancient Chinese therapies.

The earliest recording of a therapy in the form that Reflexology is known today is found in a tomb drawing of the Egyptians, dated 2330 BC, in which a person is shown holding the foot of another person and applying massage to the sole of the foot. Over the years, it has been discovered that Reflexology was known to some of the primitive tribes of Africa and also to the Red Indians. More recently, the two people responsible for documenting Reflexology as it is now known were Dr William Fitzgerald and Mrs Eunice Ingham.

Zone Therapy

Around 1913, the American Ear, Nose and Throat consultant, Dr William Fitzgerald began offering a form of treatment which was later to be termed zone therapy. Dr Fitzgerald had become interested in pressure therapies having read the works of several European doctors involved in this area in the 1500's, and had probably become acquainted with these works whilst he was practising in Vienna. Dr Fitzgerald had noticed that when treating different patients for the same disorder with a minor operation, some would feel considerable pain and others would feel very little pain. His investigations revealed that those who felt very little pain were actually producing an anaesthetic effect on themselves by applying pressure to areas of their body, or in some cases, Dr Fitzgerald himself had applied pressure to certain areas of the patient's body which produced an anaesthetic effect. By developing this work further, Dr Fitzgerald was able to describe a system of ten zones in the body, and the importance of these was that within each zone there was an energy link between certain areas, allowing one area to affect another in the same zone. Hence, by applying pressure to an area in the same zone as the ear, an anaesthetic effect could be produced in the ear. Unknowingly, in everyday life, people apply the theory of zone therapy by such actions as gritting their teeth when in pain (applying pressure to the zones of the teeth) and grasping the sides of a chair, for example at the dentist's, to try and ease pain (applying pressure to the zones of the hands).

The Zones of the Body

Dr Fitzgerald described how the body could be divided into ten longitudinal zones. (See figure 1).

If you imagine a line drawn through the centre of the body, there are five zones on either side of this median line. Each zone relates to the digits (fingers and toes) of the body: zone one extending from the thumb, up the arm to the brain and then down to the big toe; zone two extends from the second finger, up the arm to the brain and down to the second toe; zone three extends from the third finger up the arm to the brain and down to the third toe; zone four extends from the fourth finger up the arm to the brain and down to the fourth toe and zone five extends from the little finger up the arm to the brain and down to the little toe. These longitudinal zones are of equal width and extend right through

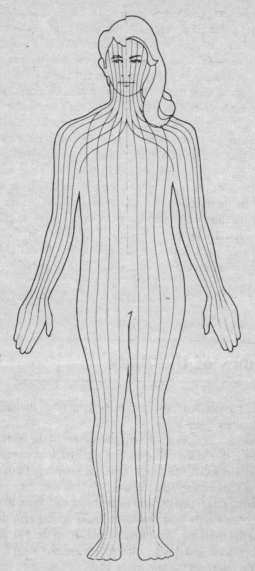

Figure 1   The longitudinal zones of the body

the body from front to back. They are like segments of the body and are not fine lines like the acupuncture meridian lines. The line marking between each zone would extend from the web of the finger to the web of the toe. Although the above description shows the zone as extending from the finger up to the brain and down to the toe, the description could be given the reverse way as from toe to finger. The importance of the ten longitudinal zones extending throughout the body is that whichever parts of the body are found within a certain zone, these parts will be linked to one another by the energy flow within the zone and can therefore affect one another. An example of this is found with kidney problems which may result in eye problems due to the fact that the kidneys and eyes are situated within the same zones. (See figure 2).

The application of zone therapy meant that it was possible to treat the various parts of the body by applying pressure to accessible areas situated within the same zone. Dr Fitzgerald used all sorts of instruments to apply pressure, such as clothes pegs, metal combs, elastic bands and metal probes. The clothes pegs would be placed over the finger tips, the combs clenched into the hands, elastic bands wrapped around the fingers and these would apply pressure to the zones in the hands which would in turn affect the same zone throughout the body. (See figures 3 and 4).

Although the hands and fingers were mainly used for such treatment, in some instances pressure was applied to the toes, ankles, wrists, elbows or knees. The amount of pressure applied was stated as being between 2 and 20 lbs and recommended as being used for a time interval of thirty seconds to five minutes, and in some cases longer. A warning was always given to remove the constricting item if the area became blue and massage to restore circulation to the area was recommended! This method was used to treat a wide range of disorders including headaches, eye problems, breast lumps, fibroids in the uterus and breathing difficulties. In addition to the ten longitudinal zones in the body, Dr Fitzgerald also described the existence of ten zones in the tongue and the mouth.

The findings of Dr Fitzgerald were met with a good deal of scepticism by most of his medical colleagues but some did experiment with his findings and on seeing the good results became devotees of the method. It was a medical journalist, Dr Edwin Bowers, who recommended that the method be termed Zone Therapy. This work was developed further by several American doctors including Dr George Starr White, Dr Joe

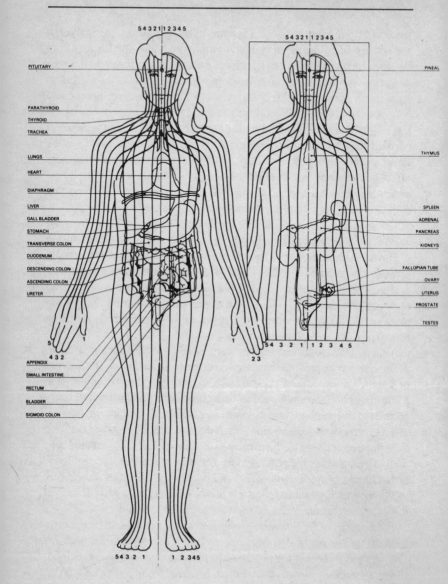

Figure 2 The zone chart

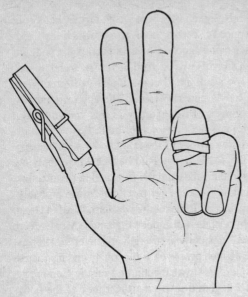

Figure 3 The use of rubber bands and clothes pegs in zone therapy

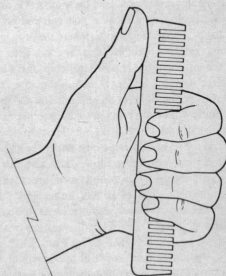

Figure 4 The use of a comb in zone therapy

Riley and his wife Elizabeth Riley, all of whom wrote further books on the subject. Dr Riley introduced the term 'hook work' which involved the hands of the practitioner being 'hooked' over a part of the body in order to manipulate the area and this was used on both tissues and joints. The theory behind hook work is still used but in a slightly different way in Reflexology. One of Dr Riley's students of Zone Therapy, Mrs Eunice Ingham, became the main pioneer of Reflexology as it is known today.

It was Eunice Ingham who was the first to describe Reflexology in its modern form. Having learnt the work of Fitzgerald and his colleagues, Mrs Ingham realized that the whole body could be treated by applying pressure to the zones found in the hands and the feet, and her two books *Stories the Feet Can Tell* and *Stories the Feet Have Told* were probably the first to be written on this subject. Reflexology was introduced to Great Britain in the early 1960's by a student of Eunice Ingham's, Mrs Doreen Bayly. Doreen Bayly showed considerable strength and determination as an elderly lady in order to enlighten people on Reflexology and instructed many of the early practitioners in Great Britain and on the Continent.

From the early work of Fitzgerald involving the zones of the body and Zone Therapy, Reflexology treatment has now evolved. Zone Therapy is still practised by some but is not so common. Although the Reflexology treatment is concentrated on the feet and sometimes the hands, there are instances where the principles of Zone Therapy are still applied. Due to the fact that the zones extend throughout the whole body, the arms and the legs are made up of the same zones. This means that a relationship will exist due to the zone connection between the right arm and the right leg and the left arm and the left leg. The joints of these limbs will bear a relation to one another and so the following are 'zone related': the hip and the shoulder; the knee and the elbow; the ankle and the wrist. Likewise, the upper leg and upper arm are zone related, and the lower leg and lower arm and also the foot and the hand. The usefulness of these 'zone related' areas will be seen at a later stage but immediately it is clear that, for example, the knee could be treated by massage to the elbow; a similar idea to the basis of 'hook work' mentioned above. These 'zone related' areas are treated in addition to the reflex areas in the feet. (See figure 5).

The longitudinal zones of the human body show the existence of an even deeper connection between the various parts of the body than the

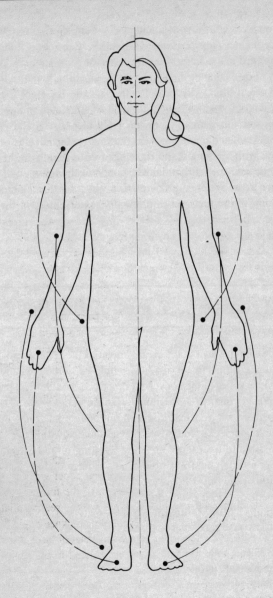

Figure 5 The zone related areas

already complex conventional biological system offers. From the findings of Eunice Ingham, it is possible to show that all the parts of the body will be represented in the feet and the hands in the same zones as they exist in the body. For example, the right kidney which is found in the body in zones two and three will have a reflex area in the right foot in zones two and three; the left kidney will have a reflex area in the left foot in zones two and three. In all cases, the right foot corresponds to the right side of the body and the left foot corresponds to the left side of the body. Similarly, with the hands, the right hand corresponds to the right side of the body and the left hand corresponds to the left side of the body. The reflex areas are arranged in such a way as to form a small picture of the body in the feet and to a slightly lesser extent in the hands.

The Transverse Zones of the Body

Before looking in detail at the arrangement of the reflex areas in the feet and the hands, a further set of zones should be introduced and these are the transverse zones of the body, first described by a German practitioner, Mrs Hanne Marquardt, who trained with Eunice Ingham. The work of Eunice Ingham showed that due to the longitudinal zones in the body and the link which existed between areas situated within the same zone, it was possible to treat these areas by working on the extremity of the zone either through the feet or the hands. Eunice Ingham had described the position of the reflex areas for all the body parts in the feet but their arrangement could be even more easily interpreted by the additional introduction of Mrs Marquardt's transverse zones. (See figure 6).

Three transverse zones can be marked on the body and these correspond to:

1 the shoulder girdle;
2 the waist;
3 the pelvic floor.

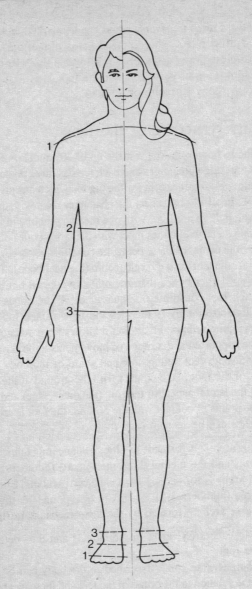

Figure 6 The transverse zones of the body

Similarly, these three transverse zones can be marked on the foot since they bear a direct relationship to the skeleton of the foot. In the hand, it is not possible to draw such a direct relationship. In order to understand the position of the transverse zones in the foot, it is first necessary to understand the bony structure of the foot.

The bony structure of the feet

Figure 7 shows how each foot is made up of 26 small bones. The bones of the toes are called phalanges and each toe has three phalanges (distal, intermediate, proximal) except for the big toe which has just two. There are therefore in all 14 phalanges: the phalanges meet with the metatarsal bones of which there are five, with one metatarsal bone in relation with each toe. The metatarsal bones meet with the tarsal bones of which there are seven − the names of these being the cuneiforms (three), the cuboid, the navicular, the talus and the calcaneum (the heel bone). The talus and calcaneum are larger bones than the other five tarsal bones. These 26 bones in each foot constitute one quarter of all the bones in the body and are held in position by 19 muscles and 107 ligaments. The structure of the foot is quite remarkable in that it allows for a considerable body weight to be supported and a range of movements to be possible. When standing with both feet taking an equal share of the body weight, the soft tissues of the foot make contact with the ground at the balls of the toes, along the lateral aspect of the sole (the outer edge) and at the heel. Between the points of contact with the ground, the foot is arched. Three distinct arches can be seen in each foot:

1 a medial arch − formed by the calcaneum, talus, navicular, cuneiforms and the medial three metatarsals (numbers 1-3),
2 a lateral arch − formed by the calcaneum, cuboid and the lateral metatarsals (numbers 4-5),
3 a transverse arch − formed by the tarso-metatarsal articulation.

The height of each arch varies in individuals and thus determines the shape of the foot.

The three transverse zones described in the body can be transposed onto the feet in relation to the bones of the feet and these can be described as follows:

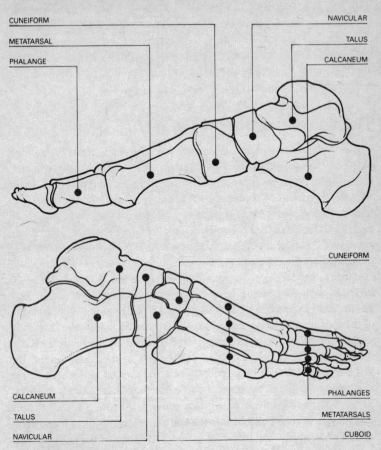

Figure 7 The bones of the foot. The medial border of the right foot is shown above and the lateral border of the right foot is shown below

1 the shoulder girdle zone relates to the region where the phalanges meet the metatarsals,
2 the waistline zone relates to the region where the metatarsals meet the tarsals,
3 the pelvic floor zone relates to the region over the tarsal bones at a level between the inner and outer malleoli (ankle bones).

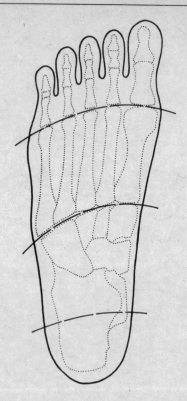

Figure 8   The transverse zones of the foot

Transverse zone one which in the body contains the areas found above the shoulder girdle and therefore includes the areas of the head and neck will relate to the areas of the foot over the phalanges, and the reflex areas to the structures of this zone will be found over the phalanges.

Transverse zone two which in the body contains the areas found below the shoulder girdle and above the waistline includes the areas of the thorax and upper abdomen, and the reflex areas to these parts will be found in the areas of the foot over the metatarsals.

Transverse zone three which in the body contains the areas found below the waistline and above the pelvic girdle includes the areas of the abdomen and pelvis, and the reflex areas to these parts will be found in the areas of the foot over the tarsals. (See figure 8).

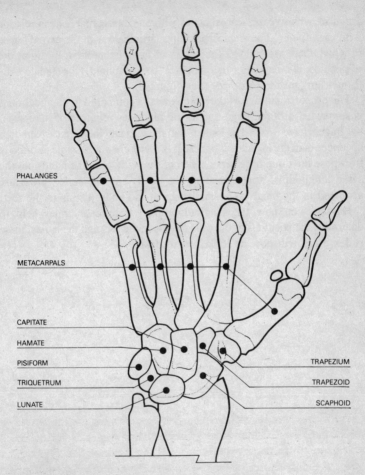

PHALANGES

METACARPALS

CAPITATE

HAMATE

PISIFORM

TRIQUETRUM

LUNATE

TRAPEZIUM

TRAPEZOID

SCAPHOID

Figure 9   The bones of the hand

The bony structure of the hands

The bones of the hands are arranged in a somewhat similar manner to those of the feet and there are 27 small bones in each hand. The bones of the fingers are also called phalanges and each finger has three phalanges except for the thumb which has just two. The phalanges articulate with five metacarpal bones with one metacarpal bone in relation with each finger. The metacarpal bones articulate with the carpal bones of which there are eight − the names of these being the trapezium, the trapezoid, the capitate, the hamate, the scaphoid, the lunate, the triquetrum and the pisiform. (See figure 9).

The proportional size of the hand bones as compared to the foot bones is somewhat different, and due to the functions required of the hands, the fingers have evolved as longer than the toes and the metacarpal bones as longer than the metatarsal bones. It is therefore not possible to directly transpose the three transverse zones of the body onto the hands but the same longitudinal zones exist in the hands and the reflex areas are arranged in the hands as a small map of the body just as in the feet.

Having seen how the longitudinal and transverse zones help to determine the positions of the reflex areas in the feet and the hands, these reflex areas will now be looked at in detail.

2 The Reflex Areas of the Feet and the Hands

The arrangement of the reflex areas in the feet and the hands is such that in whichever zone or zones of the body an organ, gland, muscle, nerve or joint is found, there will be a corresponding reflex area in the same zone or zones of the feet and in the same zone or zones of the hands.

The reflex areas of the feet and the hands will now be looked at in the order in which they are treated in a Reflexology treatment session. This order of treatment is not essential to the effectiveness of the treatment but offers a systematic pattern of covering all of the areas in the feet and the hands.

Work begins on the sole of the foot with massage to all of the reflex areas of transverse zone one, then working down the sole of the foot to massage the reflex areas of transverse zone two and then to transverse

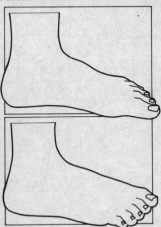

Figure 10 The different aspects of the foot. The medial (inner) aspect is shown above and the lateral (outer) aspect is shown below

zone three. The medial (inner) and lateral (outer) sides of the foot will also be massaged, and the top of the foot (see figure 10).
A similar pattern is followed when giving treatment to the hands. Normally the whole of the right foot or hand is massaged before moving on to treat the whole of the left foot or hand. Some practitioners may follow a different approach which need not affect the effectiveness of the treatment. In a treatment session, work is usually done on the feet alone but there will be occasions when the reflex areas of the hands are also incorporated or when only the reflex areas of the hands are worked on.

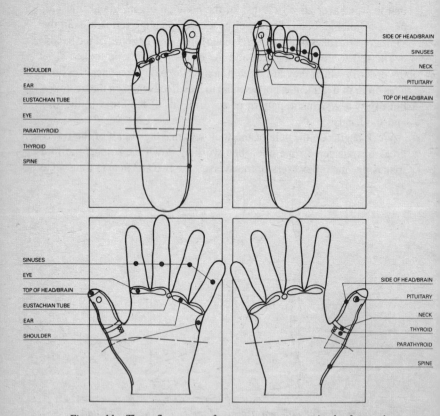

Figure 11   The reflex areas of transverse zone one in the feet and the hands

The Reflex Areas of Transverse Zone One

These reflex areas are shown in figure 11 and relate to all the parts of the body found above the shoulder girdle.

The pituitary gland

The reflex area to the pituitary gland is found roughly in the centre of the fleshy pad of the big toe in both the right and left feet. It is also found in the centre of the fleshy pad of the thumb in both the right and

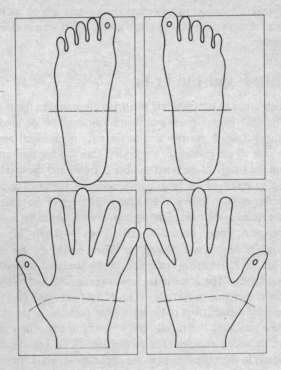

Figure 12   The reflex areas to the pituitary

left hands. In some cases, the reflex area is slightly off centre, being slightly higher or lower or more to the left or the right. (See figure 12).

The pituitary gland is found in the brain and is only about the size of a pea. It is sometimes called the master gland of the body since it controls the functions of the other endocrine (hormonal) glands in the body. The gland produces a number of different hormones which influence the activities of the thyroid gland, the adrenal glands, the kidneys, the reproductive glands, the breast and uterine muscles in pregnancy and pre-puberty development. Other functions can also be attributed to the gland.

This reflex area will be helpful in any condition where there is an imbalance of the hormonal system. Since the hormonal system is extremely sensitive and easily thrown slightly out of balance, this reflex area is found to be tender in very many cases where it need not necessarily indicate a serious problem. It is also a useful reflex area in cases of fever and insomnia.

The head and the brain

The reflex areas to the head and the brain are found in the big toes and in the thumbs. Each big toe and thumb can itself be divided into five longitudinal zones corresponding to the five longitudinal zones found on each side of the midline of the body. Thus the big toes and thumbs represent the whole of the head and brain areas, and the small toes and fingers also relate to the longitudinal zones of the head and brain.

The reflex areas to the top of the head and the top of the brain (cerebral lobes) are found in the pads of the big toes and thumbs in the area from the tip of the toe or finger, behind the nail, down the toe or finger over the distal phalanx (end bone). Down the lateral border of the big toes or thumbs are the reflex areas to the sides of the head and sides of the brain (temporal lobes). The areas in the lower part of the pad of the big toes or thumbs correspond to the reflex areas of the cerebellum (see figure 13). On the dorsal surface (top) of the big toes or thumbs are the reflex areas to the face including the mouth, the nose, the throat, the teeth and all of the surrounding muscles. The medial side of the big toes or thumbs corresponds to the reflex areas in the upper spine, and around the base of the big toes or thumbs are the reflex areas to the neck (as in figure

14). Rotation of the big toe or thumb is equivalent to rotation of the neck.

The brain, together with the spinal cord, makes up the central nervous system of the body and is therefore the major part of the control and communication system of the body. The cerebrum of the brain controls functions such as movement, hearing, vision, understanding, skin and muscle sensations and the different areas of the cerebrum have been found

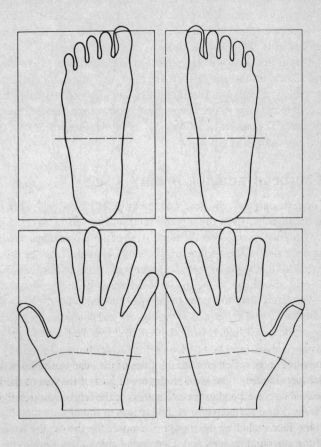

Figure 13   The reflex areas to the sides and top of the head and brain

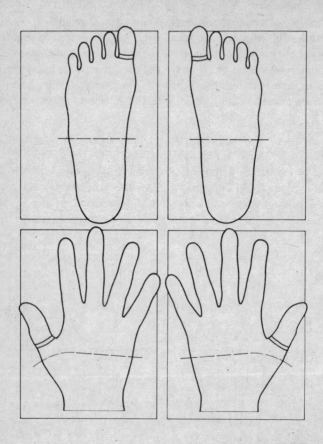

Figure 14   The reflex areas to the neck

to be associated with these different functions. The cerebellum, which is the largest part of the hind brain, coordinates movement and is also involved with the maintenance of balance. The whole of the brain area is covered and protected by the skull bones.

The reflex areas of the head and brain will be important in any condition where there is damage to the brain such as in a stroke or Parkinson's disorder. These areas will also be important when a person suffers from headaches or migraines. Because of the important control system of the brain which acts like a highly complex computer, the reflex areas will also be involved when the areas they control are affected as, for example, with sight problems, hearing problems and some muscular problems.

The spine

It has already been stated that the reflex areas to the top of the spine are found along the medial border of the big toes or thumbs. The remaining reflex areas to the spine are found along the medial sides of the feet or the hands. Referring to figure 15, the reflex areas to the cervical spine are found along the medial side between the first and second joints (A) of the big toes or thumbs; the reflex areas to the thoracic spine are found along the medial border of the first metatarsal or first

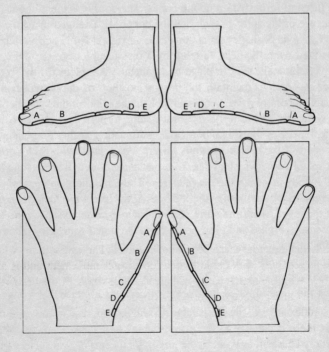

Figure 15   The reflex areas to the spine

metacarpal bones (B); the reflex areas to the lumbar spine are found along the medial border of the first cuneiform bones and distal half of the navicular bones or medial border of the trapezium bones (C); the reflex areas to the sacrum are found along the proximal half of the medial border of the navicular bones and medial part of the talus bones or along the medial border of the scaphoid bone (D); the reflex areas to the coccyx are found along the medial border of the distal third of the calcaneum or along the medial border of the styloid process of the radius (E).

The spine is made up of 33 bony segments called vertebrae. The different regions of the spine (see figure 16), from the top, are called the cervical spine (seven vertebrae the first two being named the atlas and the axis), the thoracic spine (twelve vertebrae), the lumbar spine (five vertebrae), the sacral spine of sacrum (five vertebrae), and the coccyx (four vertebrae). The vertebrae of the sacrum and the coccyx are fused to form two immobile bones. The coccyx is the tailbone. The structure of the spine is such that the bones are arranged in such a way as to give an S-shape to the spine, (as in figure 16). Each vertebra is separated from the next vertebra by a disc made out of cartilage, and the vertebrae are held in place by ligaments. Although firmly fixed in place in order to maintain the upright position of the human body, a certain amount of movement is possible in the joints of the spine between the vertebrae. The spine or vertebral column forms a thick curved column which encloses the spinal cord, the continuation of the brain stem and thus part of the central nervous system. Associated with each vertebra is a spinal nerve which arises from the spinal cord and affects the level of the body at which the nerve arises. Thus, the thoracic nerves affect the regions of the thorax, the lumbar nerves affect the lower abdomen and the legs. All of the pairs of spinal nerves receive sensations from the sensory organs and in response from the spinal cord, they then relay motor instructions to the muscles and glands involved.

The spinal reflex areas will obviously be of great importance when there is a direct back pain but may also be involved on other occasions when the area supplied by the spinal nerve is affected.

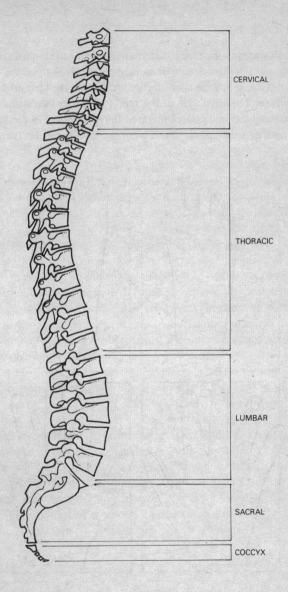

CERVICAL

THORACIC

LUMBAR

SACRAL

COCCYX

Figure 16   The curvature of the spine

The face

The reflex area to the face is found on the top of the big toes or thumbs. (See figure 17). This area will include reflex areas to all the structures of the face including the eyes, the nose, the teeth, the lips and the muscles of the face. The right side of the face is represented on the right foot or hand and the left side of the face is represented on the left foot or hand and as seen above, the big toe or thumb can be considered as

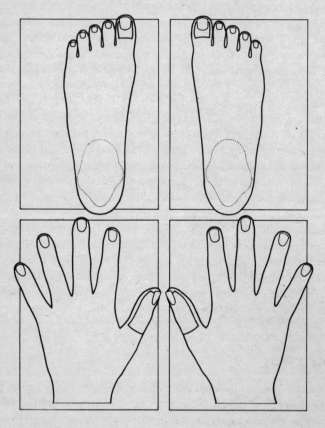

Figure 17   The reflex areas to the face

containing five longitudinal zones relating to the five longitudinal zones of the head. Other reflex areas to these parts will also be found in their corresponding zone of the foot and will be described later.

This reflex area will be important for any problem involving the face and the structures within it, including neuralgia, colds, toothache and skin problems such as acne.

The sinuses

The reflex areas to the sinuses are found in the toes and in the fingers. These reflex areas are found all the way up the back of the second, third, fourth and fifth toes or fingers and also up the sides of these toes or fingers. (See figure 18). A reflex area may also be found to these regions and to the nose on the top of the big toe or thumb. Depending on which zone or zones of the sinuses are affected, the corresponding zone or zones of the sinus reflex areas will be involved.

The sinuses are air-filled cavities formed by the bones of the front of the skull. They act as a protection for the eyes and the brain and also give resonance to the voice. They are situated above and to the sides of the nose in the cheekbones and behind the eyebrows and they communicate with the nasal cavities. Any infection from the nose can easily pass to the sinuses but it is more difficult for infections to be drained out since the exit pathways are small and can easily become congested. The mucus formed by catarrh and colds is often an indication of congestion elsewhere in the body and must be cleared to help the system to become more free of toxins.

The reflex areas to the sinuses will be important with sinus trouble, catarrh, colds, hay fever and other allergic responses of the nose and some forms of headache.

The eyes

The reflex areas to the eyes are found on the soles of the feet or palms of the hand just beneath the second and third toes or fingers. In some instances, the reflex areas may extend up these toes or fingers to a slight extent (as in figure 19). The reflex area to the right eye is found in the

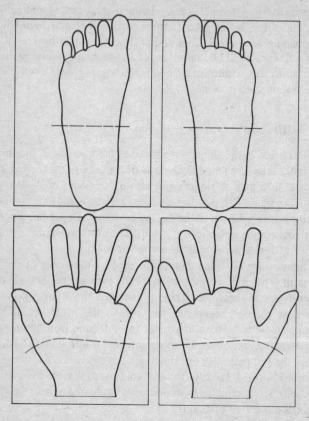

Figure 18 The reflex areas to the sinuses

right foot or hand and the reflex area to the left eye is found in the left foot or hand.

The eyes have a structure whereby they are able to transmit the light rays received from the surroundings to the brain, and the brain then interprets these impulses into visual messages which can be understood and reacted to by the body.

The lens of the eye is suspended by ligaments, and in front of the lens is a watery fluid with the front wall of this chamber formed by the cornea.

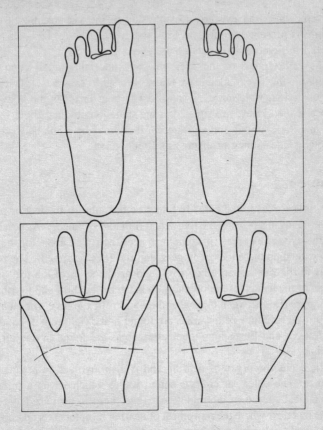

Figure 19 The reflex areas to the eyes

At the margins of the cornea are layers of cells called the conjunctiva which form the inner layer of the eyelid.

Behind the lens is a more viscous fluid, and the innermost layer of the back of the chamber containing this is the retina. The retina is the light sensitive part of the eye which converts the light rays into electrical impulses which are relayed to the brain via the optic nerve.

The colour of the eyes is determined by the pigment cells of the iris and the central aperture of this pigmented disc is called the pupil.

Movements of the eye are possible due to the various muscles and ligaments present and the eyes are protected by the eyelids. The tears are the self-cleansing agents of the eyes.

The reflex areas of the eyes will be important for all conditions involving the eyes, including faulty eyesight, cataracts, glaucoma, conjunctivitis, watering eyes and blocked tear ducts. In the body, the eyes and the kidneys are situated in the same longitudinal zones (zones two and three) and in some instances, there may be a link between eye problems and kidney problems, and vice versa.

The ears

The reflex areas to the ears are found on the soles of the feet or palms of the hands just beneath the fourth and fifth toes or fingers. As described for the eye reflex areas, in some instances the reflex areas for the ears may extend up these toes or fingers slightly. (See figure 20). The reflex areas to the Eustachian tubes are found on the soles of the feet or the palms of the hands just below the web between the third and fourth toes or fingers (i.e. between the eye and the ear reflex areas). The right ear and Eustachian tube reflex areas are found in the right foot or hand and the left ear and Eustachian tube reflex areas are found in the left foot or hand.

The ear is the organ of hearing and is also involved in maintaining balance. The outer ear collects sound waves which set up a series of mechanical stimuli in the middle ear, and these in turn are passed on to the inner ear where the movement of hearing receptors sets up impulses in the auditory nerve which passes to the auditory centre of the brain. The middle ear consists of three small bones called the malleus, incus and stapes. The inner ear, in addition to the hearing receptors, consists of areas called semi-circular canals which are the non-auditory part of the ear and concerned with the sense of balance. The Eustachian tube connects the middle ear to the throat and is involved in maintaining pressure on both sides of the tympanic membrane (ear drum). It is the Eustachian tube which opens on swallowing, yawning and sneezing and may produce a 'popping' sensation in the ear as the pressures become equalized − the sensation often occuring after the ears need to become 'unblocked' for example, when flying in an aeroplane.

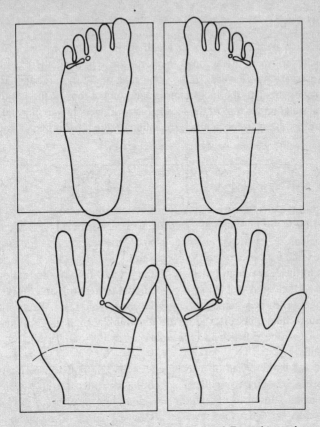

Figure 20 The reflex areas to the ears and Eustachian tubes

The reflex area of the ear is important when there are hearing problems as is the Eustachian tube reflex area. The reflex area is also important where balance is affected in conditions such as vertigo and dizziness, and the condition of tinnitus.

The teeth

The reflex areas to the teeth are found on the tops of the toes or fingers. Whichever zones of the head the teeth are found in, there will be a corresponding reflex area in the same zone of the foot or hand. Hence, the reflex areas to the incisors are found on the tops of the big toes or thumbs and on the tops of the second toes or fingers (zones one and two); the reflex areas to the canines are found on the tops of the second toes

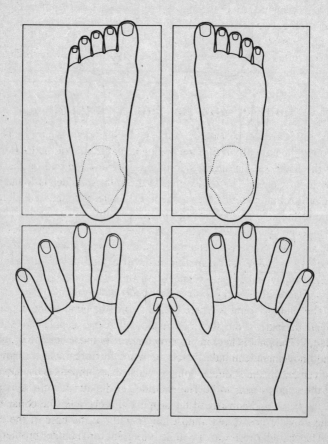

Figure 21   The reflex areas to the teeth

or fingers (zone two); the reflex areas to the premolars are found on the tops of the third toes or fingers (zone three); the reflex areas to the molars are found on the tops of the fourth toes or fingers (zone four) and the reflex areas to the wisdom teeth are found on the tops of the fifth toes or fingers (zone five). (See figure 21).

The teeth are involved in the first stages of digestion and act with the tongue, cheeks, lips and lower jaw to masticate the food and help break it down, mixing it with saliva to form a mass suitable for swallowing. The permanent teeth of the human are 16 in each jaw with two incisors, one canine, two premolars, and three molars (the third being a wisdom tooth) in each half of each jaw.

The reflex areas to the teeth may be helpful in relieving toothache or pain in the surrounding areas of the gums and jaws.

The shoulder and the shoulder girdle

The reflex area to the shoulder joint and its surrounding muscles is found around the base of the fifth toe or finger on the sole of the foot or palm of the hand, on the lateral side of the foot or hand and on the top of the foot or hand. The reflex area to the right shoulder is found in the right foot and the reflex area to the left shoulder is found in the left foot. The reflex area to the shoulder girdle extends across all five zones in both feet on the sole and on the top of the foot. As previously described, the shoulder girdle is a demarcation area between transverse zones one and two, and the reflex area to this will extend down into transverse zone two over the distal (upper) half of the metatarsal or metacarpal bones. (See figure 22).

The shoulder joint is where the humerus (the bone of the upper arm) meets the part of the shoulder girdle called the scapula (the shoulder blade). The joint is held in place by ligaments and surrounding muscles and movement can take place in many different ways. However, movement of the shoulder joint is usually accompanied by movement of other joints near to it. The shoulder girdle attaches the upper limb to the trunk and consists of the scapula and clavicle (the collar bone). The clavicle lies across almost horizontally at the base of the neck.

The shoulder reflex area will be important for shoulder problems and nearly always the shoulder girdle reflex area will also be involved as

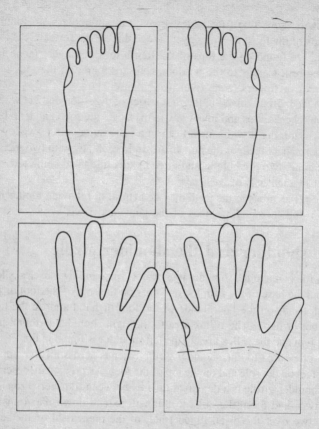

Figure 22   The reflex areas to the shoulders

will the reflex area to the neck. Problems with the arm may also be related to shoulder and neck problems.

The upper arm

(Although not present in the first transverse zone of the body, the reflex area to the upper arm will be discussed here following on from the shoulder joint reflex area after which it will normally be massaged).

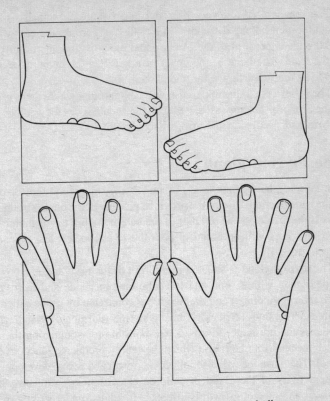

Figure 23 The reflex areas to the arms and elbows

The reflex area to the upper arm is found on the outer border of the foot or hand slightly to the top of the foot or hand. The right arm will be represented on the right foot or hand and the left arm will be represented on the left foot or hand. The area is found leading down from the shoulder reflex area along the outer edge of the fifth metatarsal or metacarpal bone on the side and top of the foot or hand. The reflex area to the elbow joint is found at the base of the outer edge of the fifth metatarsal bone which projects slightly on the side of the foot or along the metacarpal bone at waist level on the hand. (See figure 23).

The arm is also referred to as the upper limb and consists of the shoulder joint linking the upper limb to the body trunk, the elbow joint linking the upper arm to the forearm and the wrist linking the forearm to the hand. The bone of the upper arm is called the humerus and the bones of the forearm are the radius and ulna.

The reflex area to the upper arm will be important where there is pain in the arm or problems associated with the shoulder or elbow joints such as pins and needles in the arm, or tennis elbow.

The thyroid gland

The thyroid gland reflex area is found in the sole of the foot or palm of the hand over the base of the proximal phalanx of the big toe or thumb. This is the area over the top half of the ball of the big toe or thumb and the reflex area will be found in both the right and left feet or hands. (See figure 24).

The thyroid gland is situated in the root of the neck and is a bow-tie shaped gland with a right and left lobe on either side and in front of the trachea (windpipe) and the two lobes connected by tissue called the isthmus. The thyroid gland is an endocrine (hormonal) gland which produces the hormone, thyroxine, responsible for stimulating the rate of cell metabolism (the rate at which the energy-producing functions take place). The hormone will also influence growth and sexual development. Underactivity of the gland in children can result in cretinism where physical and mental growth is affected. In adults, underactivity of the gland produces a condition known as myxoedema where there is weight gain, puffiness of the face and eyelids and a general slowing down of the metabolic processes resulting in weakness, tiredness and other symptoms. It is the thyroid gland which people refer to when they say that a weight problem is 'glandular' though often the problem may not be directly glandular but affected by food intake in excess of food needs! With an overactive gland, a condition known as thyrotoxicosis, all the body processes are speeded up with resultant restlessness, nervousness, irritability, loss of weight, increased perspiration all being possible symptoms. In addition, the gland itself may swell and the eyes protrude – the latter being an obvious indication of an overactive gland. An enlargement of the thyroid gland is galled a goitre. The thyroid gland

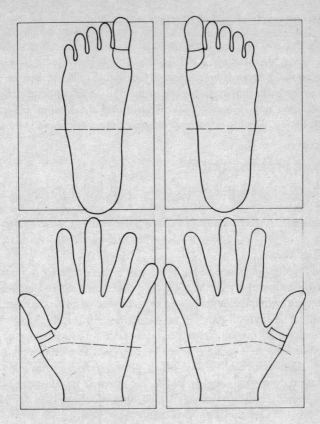

Figure 24   The reflex areas to the thyroid

also produces a hormone called calcitonin which acts to lower the level of the mineral calcium in the blood.

With Reflexology treatment, the effect is one of balance so that the same treatment will be necessary whether the gland be over or under active.

The reflex area to the thyroid gland will be helpful to imbalances of the thyroid and may also be involved with other glandular imbalances particularly those involving the reproductive glands.

The parathyroid glands

The reflex areas to the parathyroid glands are found associated with the reflex areas to the thyroid gland. The right upper parathyroid gland reflex is found in the upper lateral region of the thyroid reflex area in the upper part of the ball of the right big toe or thumb; the left upper parathyroid gland reflex area is found similarly positioned in the ball of the left big toe or thumb. The lower parathyroid reflex areas are found in the lower

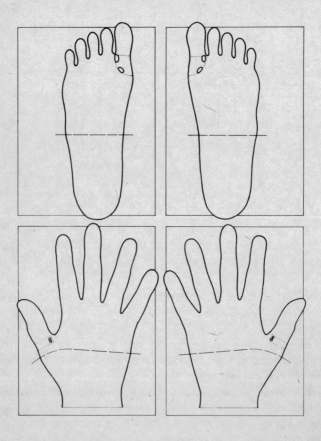

Figure 25   The reflex areas to the parathyroids

lateral margins of the thyroid reflex areas in the right and left feet or hands. (See figure 25).

The parathyroid glands are found as four small glands embedded in the back of the thyroid gland in the neck. On both the right and left sides there is an upper and a lower gland. The parathyroid glands are endocrine glands and produce a hormone called parathormone which influences the calcium level in the blood. This hormone is able to increase the level of calcium in the blood by acting on the kidneys to decrease calcium excretion and by acting on the bones to cause calcium to be given up from the bone stores. The function of parathormone is opposed by that of calcitonin from the thyroid so that between these two hormones, blood calcium level is maintained at a balanced level necessary for the correct functioning of nerves and muscles. If there is a decrease in the amount of parathormone produced, the blood calcium level falls and the condition of tetany can result where there is spontaneous and prolonged twitching of muscles. If there is an increase in the amount of parathormone produced, the blood calcium level rises with increased calcium being taken from the bones making them soft and brittle.

The parathyroid reflex areas will be helpful in conditions where the calcium level of the blood is affected such as muscle twitching and spasms, kidney stones, brittle bones and some arthritic and rheumatic conditions.

The Reflex Areas of Transverse Zone Two

These reflex areas are shown in figure 26 and relate to all the parts of the body found between the shoulder girdle and waist level.

The lungs

The reflex areas to the lungs are found in all five zones of the sole of the foot or the hand in the area over the upper half of the metatarsal or metacarpal bones. The reflex area of the right lung is found in the right foot or hand and the reflex area of the left lung is found in the left foot or hand. The reflex areas to the trachea (windpipe) and the

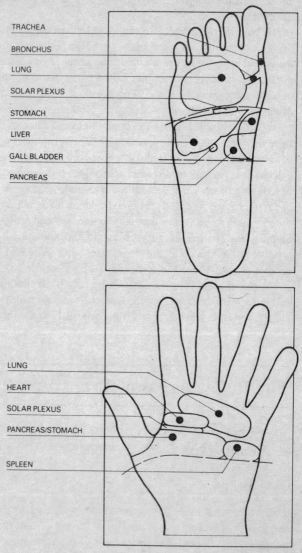

TRACHEA
BRONCHUS
LUNG
SOLAR PLEXUS
STOMACH
LIVER
GALL BLADDER
PANCREAS

LUNG
HEART
SOLAR PLEXUS
PANCREAS/STOMACH
SPLEEN

*Figure 26 The reflex areas of transverse zone two in the feet
and the hands*

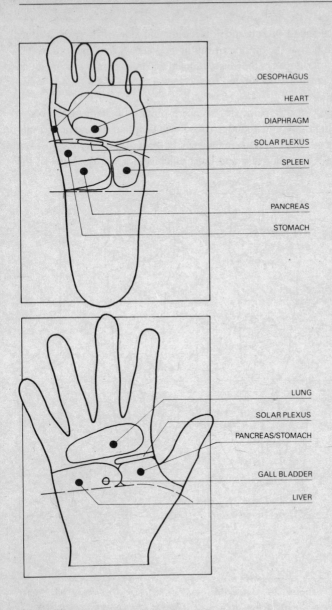

OESOPHAGUS

HEART

DIAPHRAGM

SOLAR PLEXUS

SPLEEN

PANCREAS

STOMACH

LUNG

SOLAR PLEXUS

PANCREAS/STOMACH

GALL BLADDER

LIVER

bronchi are found in zone one on the medial side of the foot leading down from below the big toe or thumb and across into the lung reflex area. The reflex areas to the lungs, bronchi and trachea may also be found in similar positions on the top of the feet or back of the hands (as in figure 27).

The lungs are the main part of the respiratory system of the body. Air taken in through the mouth passes down the pharynx and larynx into the trachea which is situated in the neck in front of the oesophagus. The trachea leads into the right and left bronchus at about the level of the

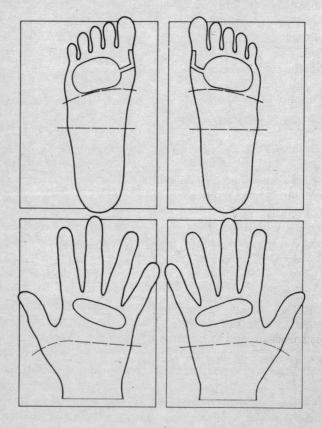

Figure 27 The reflex areas to the lungs, bronchi and trachea

fourth thoracic vertebra. The two main bronchi divide into smaller and smaller tubes called bronchioles and these end as alveolar ducts from which spring clusters of thin-walled air sacs called alveoli. The structure of the lungs is thus often described as 'tree-like'. The right lung is made up of three lobes with the left lung having only two lobes. Two thin layers called pleura cover the lungs. The lungs occupy the whole of the thoracic cavity with the tops of the lungs passing up behind the clavicles, and the base of the lungs resting on the diaphragm. The alveoli are the areas through which the exchange of gases takes place, with oxygen being given up to the blood to be carried around the body and carbon dioxide being taken up from the blood by the lungs to be expelled.

With all breathing problems, the reflex areas of the lungs will be important and this will include such conditions as asthma, bronchitis, emphysema and pleurisy.

The sternum and the ribs

The reflex areas to the sternum are found on the top of the foot or hand in zone one on the medial edge of the head of the first metatarsal or metacarpal bone in both the right and left foot or right or left hand. (See figure 28).

The reflex areas to the ribs are found in both feet or hands across all five zones over the metatarsal or metacarpal bones and therefore overlap the reflex areas to the lungs on both the sole and top of the foot or palm and back of the hand.

The sternum (breastbone) is situated in the front of the body in a central position in the upper thorax.

There are 12 pairs of ribs which form the sides of the chest area and the first seven pairs (true ribs) are joined to the sternum; the lower five pairs are not attached to the sternum (false ribs). The eighth, ninth and tenth pairs are joined by cartilage to the seventh pair and the eleventh or twelfth pairs are not attached at the front and are often referred to as 'floating' ribs. On inspiration, the ribs and sternum move upwards and outwards to increase the width of the chest and on expiration the ribs and sternum move downwards and inwards to diminish the width of the chest. These areas are therefore an important part of the respiratory process.

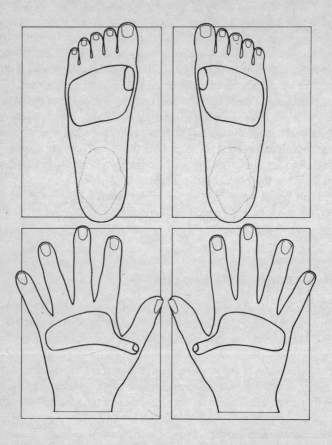

Figure 28   The reflex areas to the sternum and ribs

The reflex areas to the sternum and ribs will be important where there is direct damage to these areas and in some breathing disorders.

The diaphragm

The reflex areas to the diaphragm are found in both feet and both hands. In the sole of the foot, the level of the reflex area corresponds to a line

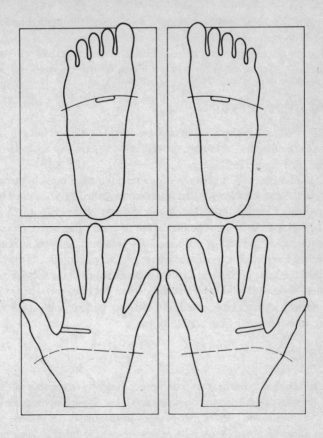

Figure 29 The reflex areas to the diaphragm and solar plexus

across from the lower area of the ball of the big toe which is in some cases more evident due to a well developed transverse arch to the foot. In the hands the level of the reflex area to the diaphragm can be drawn across the palm of the hand from just above the web between the thumb and second finger. (See figure 29).

The diaphragm is a large, muscular, dome-shaped wall which separates the thorax from the abdomen. It is involved in the process of respiration: on breathing in, the diaphragm contracts and descends to increase the depth of the chest and on breathing out, the diaphragm relaxes and ascends to decrease the depth of the chest.

Due to its involvement in respiration, the diaphragm will be an important reflex area with many problems of respiration.

The solar plexus

The reflex areas to the solar plexus are found at the level of the reflex areas to the diaphragm in both the feet and the hands in zones two and three. (See figure 29).

The solar plexus is a network of nerves giving off branches to many parts of the abdominal cavity and is sometimes called the abdominal brain. It is situated behind the stomach and in front of the diaphragm.

The reflex areas to the solar plexus are of great value where relaxation is required. At the end of a Reflexology treatment session, a relaxing breathing exercise is carried out where pressure is applied to the reflex areas to the solar plexus and as the patient breathes in the feet are gently pushed towards the body and as the patient breathes out, the pressure on the reflex areas is released and the feet pulled gently back. This exercise is repeated four or five times.

The heart

The reflex area to the heart is found predominantly in the sole of the left foot or palm of left hand in zones two and three above diaphragm level in the foot or hand and over the metatarsal or metacarpal bones of these zones. It may also be possible to find a reflex area to the heart in zone one of the left foot or hand at the same level since in the body the heart is present in zone one but the heart reflex area is a slight exception to the standard rule of finding the reflex areas in exactly the same zones of the feet or hands as to the zones where an organ is found in the body. (See figure 30).

In the body the heart is found in the region of the thoracic cavity in a central position with two-thirds of the heart to the left side of the mid-line and one third of the heart to the right side. It is a conical shaped muscular organ with the base of the heart positioned upwards and backwards and the apex of the heart positioned downwards and forwards to the left. The heart can be divided into four chambers, two on either

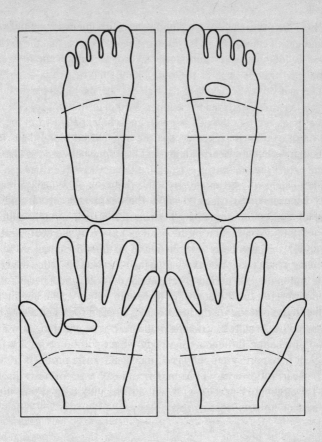

Figure 30 The reflex areas to the heart

side of a dividing middle line called the septum. The upper chambers of the heart are called the right and left atria and the lower chambers of the heart are called the right and left ventricles. The function of the heart is to pump the blood around the body and this is achieved by a cycle of rhythmic contractions and relaxations of the heart muscle. Oxygenated blood leaves the left side of the heart from left atrium to left ventricle and into the aorta (the largest blood vessel in the body). This blood then travels through a system of arteries and arterioles until reaching the tissues where the blood vessels become very narrow-walled vessels called capillaries. It is within the capillary beds that the exchange of gases, food and waste substances takes place and the de-oxygenated blood then travels back to the right side of the heart via a system of venules and veins. Returning to the right atrium, the blood passes through the right ventricle and then to the lungs. Within the pulmonary circulation of the lungs, carbon dioxide is given up to be expelled from the lungs and more oxygen is picked up and the oxygenated blood then returns to the left side of the heart. To prevent backflow between the chambers of the heart, certain valves exist called the aortic valve (between aorta and left ventricle), the pulmonary valve (between pulmonary artery and right ventricle), the tricuspid valve (between right atrium and right ventricle) and the mitral valve (between left atrium and left ventricle). The rhythmic contraction of the heart is known as the heart beat and, in general, the heart beats between 60 and 80 times per minute. The cycle of events which take place every time the heart beats is called the cardiac cycle and involves a period of relaxation (diastole) and a period of contraction (systole) and the closure of certain valves at the beginning of each of these periods are the heart sounds listened for when taking blood pressure. The healthy functioning of the heart is essential to allow a good blood circulation throughout the body which will be necessary for an efficient transport system of gases, foods and waste products to occur.

The heart reflex area will be important in all cases of heart disorders and for circulatory problems. It will also be important where there is a raised or lowered blood pressure.

The thymus

The reflex area to the thymus is found in both the right and left feet or hands in zone one in an area over the medial half of the ball of the big toe in the sole of the foot or ball of the thumb in the palm of the hand. (See figure 31).

The thymus gland is situated in the thoracic cavity close to the heart. It is important before the age of puberty in aiding the development of the body's immune system. After puberty, the size of the gland decreases and the exact function of the thymus in the adult is undecided though it may still be involved in the immune system.

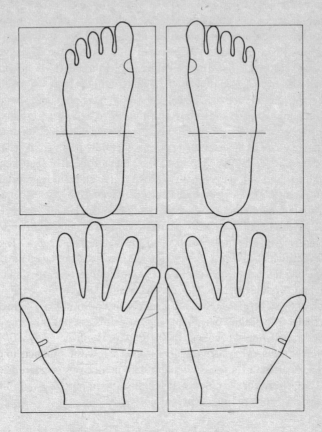

Figure 31   The reflex areas to the thymus

The reflex area to the thymus is important before the age of puberty when the immune system does not function correctly and possibly may help in conditions in the adult where the immune system is affected.

The liver

The reflex area to the liver is found in only the right foot or hand in the sole of the foot or palm of the hand. It is found predominantly in zones

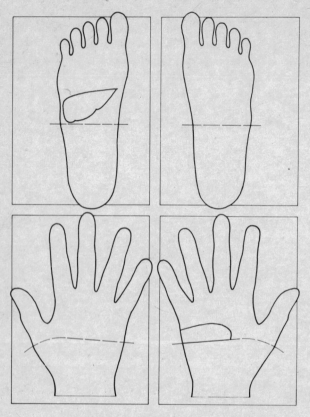

Figure 32   The reflex areas to the liver

three, four and five below the diaphragm level but above waist level
and will be present over the lower half of the metatarsal or metacarpal
bones. (See figure 32).

The liver is the largest gland in the body and it is found in all five
zones on the right side of the body above waist level and also extends
slightly over the left side of the body in zones one and two. It has many
different functions and these include the manufacture of bile, a substance
required for the digestion of fats; the storage of sugars in the form of

glycogen which can be used when the body needs an increased supply of energy; the detoxification of toxic materials absorbed by the body; the storage and metabolism of fats and proteins.

The liver reflex is important where there is jaundice, hepatitis, problems with fat digestion or conditions where there is increased toxicity in the body.

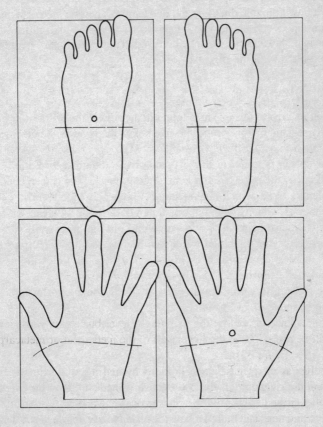

Figure 33 The reflex areas to the gall bladder

The gall bladder

The reflex area to the gall bladder is found in the right foot or hand in the sole of the foot or palm of the hand in zone three just above waist level. The reflex area is closely associated to that of the liver. (See figure 33).

The gall bladder is a small, muscular, pear-shaped sac found in the body attached to the under surface of the right lobe of the liver. Its function is to store the bile manufactured by the liver and the presence of fats in the duodenum of the small intestine causes a substance to be released which in turn stimulates the gall bladder to contract and release its stores of bile down the bile duct into the duodenum. The bile then acts on the fat substances present to allow them to be absorbed and utilized.

The gall bladder reflex will be involved in any conditions where there is a problem with the digestion of fats.

The spleen

The reflex area to the spleen is found in the sole of the left foot or palm of the left hand in zones four and five below the level of the diaphragm and above the waist level. (See figure 34).

The spleen is found in the left side of the abdomen to the left side of the tail of the pancreas and behind the stomach. The spleen contains lymphatic tissue which manufactures the white blood cells, called lymphocytes, which are an important part of the body's defence system. The spleen also helps in the breakdown of old red blood cells and can act as a reservoir for blood which can be released into the circulation when there is a need such as in a haemorrhage or following severe muscular exertion.

The reflex area to the spleen is important in some cases of infection and in some cases of anaemia.

The pancreas

The reflex area to the pancreas is found in the soles and palms of both feet and both hands. It will be present in zones one, two and three of the left foot and hand, and in zones one and two of the right foot or hand. It is present just above waist level and over the lower thirds of the metatarsal bones of these zones. (See figure 35).

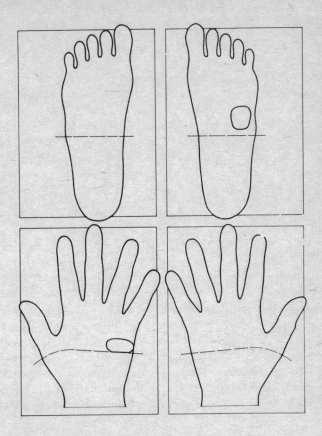

Figure 34   The reflex areas to the spleen

The pancreas in the body in found lying across the middle portions of the body above the waist and is behind the stomach. The 'tail' of the pancreas to the left lies against the spleen and the 'body' of the pancreas to the right lies in the C-shaped loop of the duodenum. The pancreas is probably best known for its function as an endocrine gland and for the production of the hormone insulin which is important in the control of sugar metabolism. Insulin is able to lower the blood sugar level. The pancreas also produces another hormone called glucagon which is again

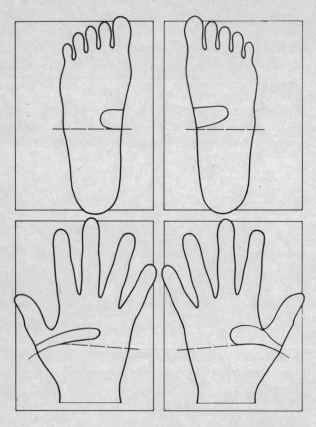

Figure 35 The reflex areas to the pancreas

involved with sugar metabolism and acts to increase the blood sugar level
by allowing the release of glycogen stores from the liver. In addition
to its hormonal functions, the pancreas is also involved in the process
of digestion. The gland produces a substance called pancreatic juice which
passes from the pancreas into the duodenum down the pancreatic duct
and this juice contains several different enzymes which can act on the
food substances to break them down into smaller-sized particles to be
more readily absorbed from the digestive tract.

The pancreas reflex area will be important where there are disturbances in sugar metabolism in such conditions as diabetes and hyper- and hypoglycaemia, and it will also be involved in certain digestive problems.

The stomach

The reflex area to the stomach is found in both the right and left feet and hands in the soles and the palms respectively. The reflex area is found in zones one, two and three on the left side and zones one on the

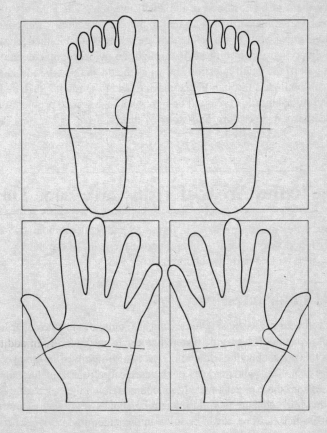

Figure 36 The reflex areas to the stomach

right side and is present below the level of the diaphragm and above the waist level. (See figure 36).

The stomach is a muscular sac lying mainly to the left side of the body just above waist level and its size and shape will vary depending on its contents and muscle tone. The stomach acts as a reservoir for the food substances eaten which enter into it down the oesophagus through the cardiac sphincter. In the stomach food is mixed with gastric juices and enzymes are present which start the digestive process. Gastric juice is rich in acid which helps kill bacteria present and affects certain minerals to allow them to be absorbed in the small intestine. The contents of the stomach are diluted or concentrated so that they are of the same concentration as the body's fluids before they are passed on to the small intestine. The emptying of the stomach is through the pyloric sphincter into the first part of the small intestine known as the duodenum. Foods such as starches will pass through the stomach quicker than foods such as fats.

The stomach reflex area will be important in digestive problems such as indigestion, heartburn and stomach ulcers.

The Reflex Areas of Transverse Zone Three

These reflex areas are shown in figure 38 and relate to the parts of the body found below waist level and above the level of the pelvic floor. This area will contain the abdominal organs.

The small intestine

The reflex areas to the small intestine are found in the soles of the feet and the palms of the hands occupying zones one, two, three and four on both the right and the left sides. This area will be over the tarsal bones of the foot and the lower part of the metacarpal bones of the hand in the region below waist level. (See figure 37).

The small intestine is a muscular tube about twenty feet or more in length which lies in a coiled position in the abdominal cavity. The first part of the small intestine is called the duodenum and this is a C-shaped

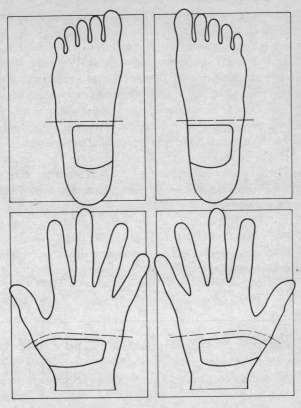

Figure 37 The reflex areas to the small intestine

tube starting just to the right of the end of the stomach and surrounding the body of the pancreas on the right side. The duodenum leads into the next part of the small intestine called the jejunum and then the small intestine becomes the part known as the ilium which is its largest part. The small intestine receives the food from the stomach and also pancreatic juice from the pancreas and bile from the gall bladder. The action of various enzymes in this region helps to break down the food substances in smaller-sized particles which can be absorbed from the digestive tract.

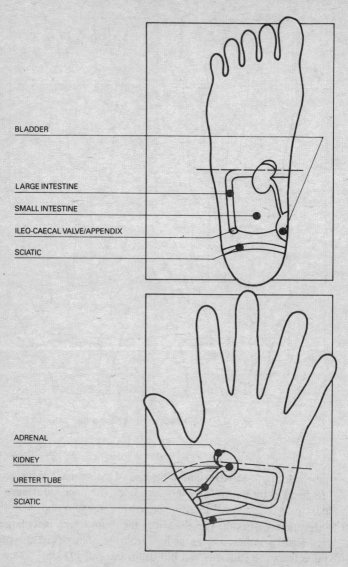

BLADDER

LARGE INTESTINE

SMALL INTESTINE

ILEO-CAECAL VALVE/APPENDIX

SCIATIC

ADRENAL

KIDNEY

URETER TUBE

SCIATIC

*Figure 38 The reflex areas of transverse zone three in the feet
and the hands*

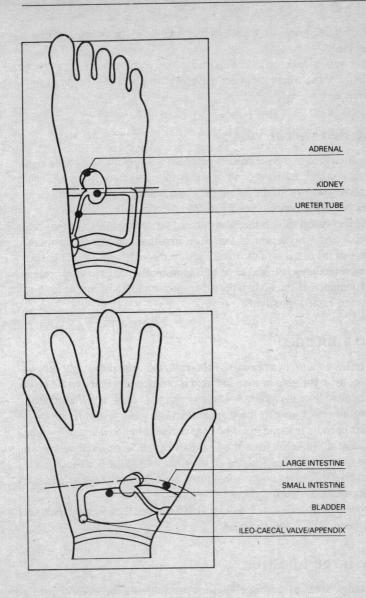

The small intestine is the main area of the digestive tract where absorption takes place.

This reflex area will be important with many digestive problems including those where there is poor breakdown and absorption of food substances.

The ileo-caecal valve

The reflex area to the ileo-caecal valve is found on the sole of the right foot or palm of the right hand in zones four and five. It is positioned just above the level of the pelvic floor and will be found over the tarsal bones or carpal bones. (See figure 39).

The ileo-caecal valve is the valve situated between the ileum of the small intestine and the caecum of the large intestine and thus controls the passage of the contents of the small intestine through to the large intestine.

This reflex area is found to be of importance in cases of constipation and conditions of the body where there is a build up of mucus such as sinus and catarrh problems.

The appendix

The reflex area to the appendix is found on the sole of the right foot or palm of the right hand in zone four and is positioned just above the level of the pelvic floor over the tarsal bones or carpal bones. It is immediately below the reflex area to the ileo-caecal valve. (As in figure 39).

The appendix is found in the body as a small blind-ended narrow tube extending downwards from the first part of the large intestine known as the caecum which is situated on the right side of the body just above the level of the pelvic floor. Although of limited significance in humans, the appendix is rich in lymphoid tissue.

The appendix reflex area is of importance when there is inflammation and obstruction in the appendix.

The large intestine

The reflex areas to the large intestine are found in the soles or palms of both feet or hands. Starting on the right foot or hand, with the caecum

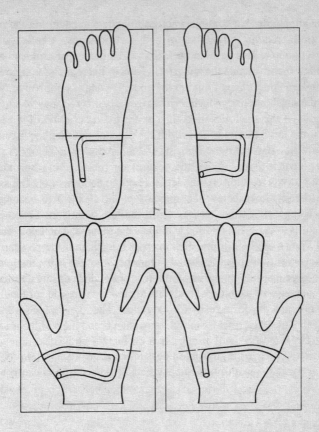

*Figure 39   The reflex areas to the large intestine, ileo-caecal valve
and appendix*

reflex found in zones four and five just above the level of the pelvic
floor over the tarsal or carpal bones, the reflex area to the ascending
colon leads up from this area to waist level. The reflex area for the
transverse colon then goes across at waist level covering all five zones
on the right and then left foot or hand. On the left foot or hand this reflex
area is continued down the zones four and five with the reflex area to
the descending colon and at a similar level to the caecum, the reflex area

to the sigmoid colon continues across to zone one ending in the reflex area to the rectum in zone one of both feet or hands. A reflex area to the rectum may also be found up the back of the leg or arm leading up for a few inches behind the ankle or in front of the wrist. (See figure 39).

The large intestine is found in the abdomen and is a long tube, wider than the small intestine, which forms three sides of a rectangle to surround the coils of the small intestine. Just as for the description of the reflex areas, the large intestine starts with the caecum and then the ascending colon which passes up the right side of the abdomen to below the liver where it bends to the left (hepatic flexure) and passes across the abdomen as the transverse colon. At the left side of the abdomen, the transverse colon bends down below the spleen (splenic flexure) to become the descending colon which passes down the left side of the abdomen. It then turns towards the midline and takes the shape of a double S-shaped bend known as the sigmoid flexure which leads into the rectum. The rectum is centrally positioned and in turn becomes the anus, the last part of the large intestine. In the large intestine, water and salts are absorbed in order to conserve the body's fluids and to present the residue of food from digestion in a dry form ready for excretion. The food residue is moved along the intestinal tract by muscle movements and the residue is stored in the large intestine until distension of the rectum stimulates elimination.

The reflex area to the large intestine is important with digestive problems and in particular with problems such as diarrhoea and constipation.

The bladder

The reflex area to the bladder is found in zone one of the foot or hand and is present in both feet and hands. It will be found on the side of the foot below the inner ankle bone and over the medial distal edge of the calcaneum bone – sometimes a slightly puffy area. Also, in some instances, there may be a reflex on the sole of the foot over the area of the talus bone. On the hand the reflex area is similarly placed on the palm of the hand and round to the back of the hand in zone one over the medial carpal bones. (See figure 40).

The bladder is a large elastic, muscular sac situated in the centre of the pelvis. It acts as a storage area for urine and is also involved with

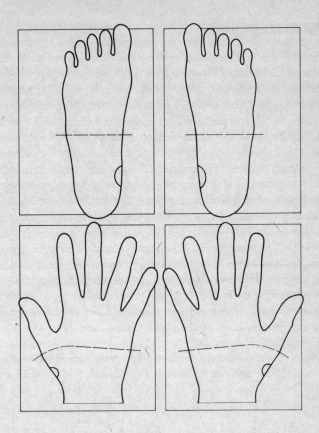

Figure 40 The reflex areas to the bladder

the expulsion of urine which will pass from the bladder down the urethra to be eliminated.

The bladder reflex area is important with all problems connected with the urinary tract and where the bladder itself is affected such as by infection, or where there is loss of control of the muscles of the bladder causing incontinence.

The ureter tube

The reflex areas to the ureter tubes are found in the soles of the feet or the palms of the hands linking the reflex area of the bladder to the reflex area of the kidney. This area is, therefore, across from zone one in the pelvic area of the foot or hand (reflex area to the bladder) leading upwards to zones two and three and approximately waist level of the foot or hand (reflex area to the kidney). The reflex area to the right ureter

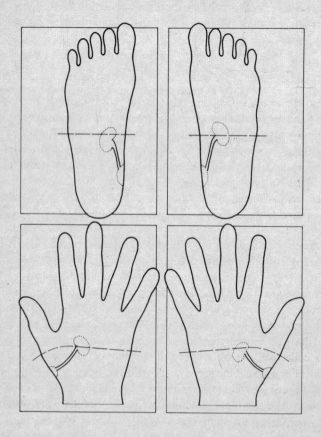

Figure 41   The reflex areas to the ureter tubes

tube is found in the right foot or hand and the reflex area to the left ureter tube is found in the left foot or hand. (See figure 41).

The ureter tube is a thin muscular tube about ten to twelve inches in length which passes downwards and medially to join the bladder. There are two ureter tubes, one from each kidney, leading into the bladder and these act merely as transport systems for the urine produced by the kidney to be carried to the bladder which is the storage area for the urine until it is eliminated.

These reflex areas are important in any condition where the urinary tract is affected such as kidney infections, bladder infections, and with kidney stones.

The kidneys

The reflex area to the kidneys is found in the sole of the foot or the palm of the hand, with the right kidney represented in the right foot or hand and the left kidney represented in the left foot or hand. The reflex area is positioned in zones two and three at approximately waist level and will be found over the metatarsal-tarsal joints in these zones or the metacarpal bones of these zones. (See figure 42).

There are two kidneys in the body which lie to the back of the abdomen at waist level with the right kidney being positioned slightly lower than the left kidney. These bean-shaped organs are about four inches long, two inches wide and one inch thick. The function of the kidneys is to separate certain waste products from the blood and therefore to maintain the blood at a constant composition. The basic unit of the kidney is called a nephron and within each kidney there are approximately one million nephrons. After a process of filtration and concentration in the kidney tubules, urine is formed which collects in the bladder. The kidneys are one of the main excretory systems of the body and the term urinary system refers collectively to the kidneys, ureter tubes, bladder and urethra.

The reflex areas to the kidneys are involved in all cases of problems with the urinary system including infections and kidney stones and may also be involved in other conditions of toxicity in the body where the kidneys are not functioning correctly as excretory organs.

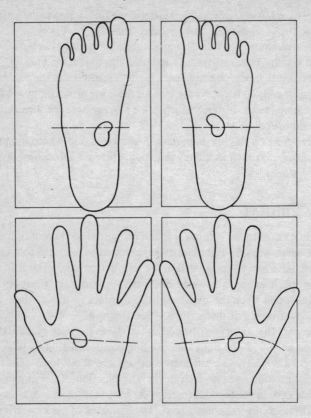

Figure 42   The reflex areas to the kidneys

The adrenal glands

The reflex area to the adrenal glands is found in the sole of the foot or palm of the hand with the right adrenal gland represented in the right foot or hand and the left adrenal gland represented in the left foot or hand. These reflex areas are very close to those of the kidneys and are found in zone two just above waist level slightly above and to the medial

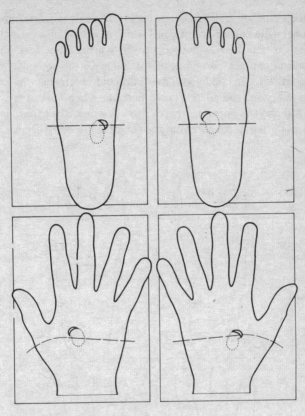

Figure 43 The reflex areas to the adrenals

side of the kidney reflexes. These reflex areas will be found over the base of the metatarsal and metacarpal bones. (See figure 43).

In the body there are two adrenal glands, one on the right and one on the left side, and these are positioned like small caps on the upper and medial part of each kidney. Although quite small glands, anatomically each gland can be divided into two distinct regions known as the adrenal cortex (outer layer) and the adrenal medulla (inner layer). The adrenal glands are part of the endocrine (hormonal) system of the body and they produce a number of different hormones. The adrenal cortex produces hormones called mineralocorticoids which affect the mineral and water balance in the body, glucocorticoids which affect carbohydrate metabolism and sex hormones which influence the secondary sexual characteristics. In addition, the corticoid hormones have anti-inflammatory and anti-allergic properties. The adrenal cortex is essential to life and plays an important role in states of stress. The adrenal medulla produces the hormones adrenalin and noradrenalin which act in a similar

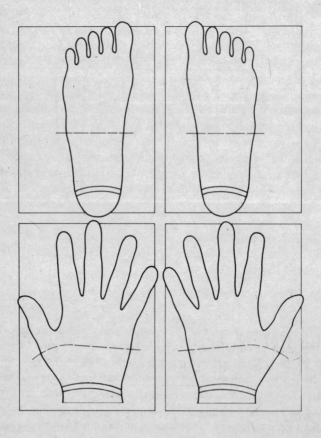

Figure 44   The reflex areas to the sciatic nerve

manner to the sympathetic nervous system by preparing the systems of the body to react efficiently in times of emergency or stress.

The reflex areas to the adrenal glands will be important in any condition where there is an imbalance of the hormonal system and in cases involving the malfunction of the kidneys. The areas will also be important in cases of inflammation (including arthritis and skin problems) and allergies and in all cases of stress.

The sciatic nerve

The reflex area to the sciatic nerve is found in both feet and both hands across the sole of the foot or across the palm of the hand. In the foot, the sciatic 'loop' is found across the calcaneum bone approximately one third of the way down the pad of the heel. This reflex area can be continued across the sides of the foot below the ankle bones and then continued up the back of the leg on either side of the Achilles tendon. In the hand, the reflex area is found across the wrist. (See figure 44).

The sciatic nerve is the largest nerve in the body and arises from the sacral plexus of nerves formed by the lower lumbar and upper sacral spinal nerves. It supplies the leg and passes from the spine, down across the buttock and down the back of the leg to divide just above the knee into two main branches which supply the lower leg. There is a right and left sciatic nerve supplying the right and left leg, respectively.

The reflex area to the sciatic nerve will be important in cases of sciatica which is a condition involving pain along the pathway of the sciatic nerve and which can have several different causes.

The Reflex Areas of the Lateral Border of the Foot or the Hand

The reflex areas of the lateral (outer) border of the foot or the hand relate to the joints of the body and their ligaments and surrounding muscles. (See figure 45).

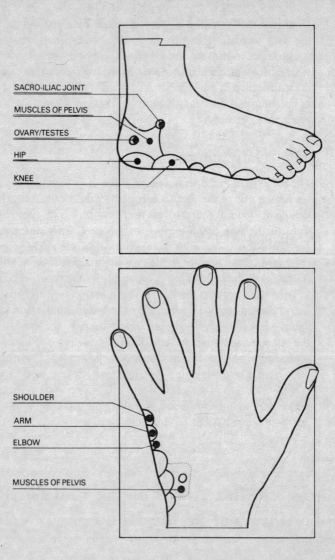

SACRO-ILIAC JOINT

MUSCLES OF PELVIS

OVARY/TESTES

HIP

KNEE

SHOULDER

ARM

ELBOW

MUSCLES OF PELVIS

Figure 45   The reflex areas of the lateral border of the feet and the hands

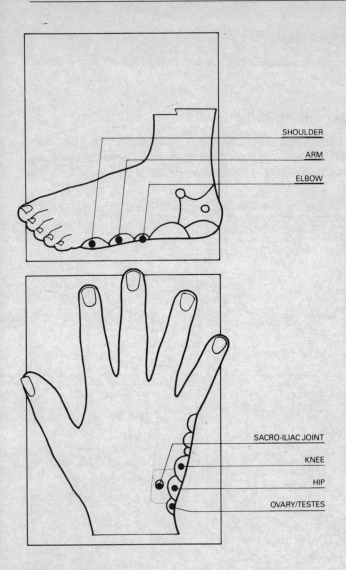

The shoulder

The reflex areas to the shoulder joint have been described on page 43.

The upper arm

The reflex areas to the upper arm and the elbow joint have been described on page 44.

The sacro-iliac joint

The reflex area to the sacro-iliac joint is found just in front of the outer malleolus (ankle bone) in a small dip about in line with the fourth toe. On the hand, the reflex area is found on the back of the hand to the lateral

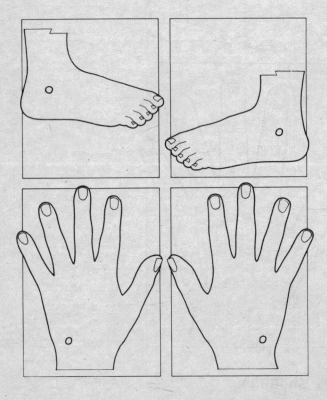

Figure 46   The reflex areas to the sacro-iliac joint

side just above the wrist. The right sacro-iliac joint is found on the right foot or hand and the left sacro-iliac joint is found on the left foot or hand. (See figure 46).

The sacro-iliac joint is where the sacrum of the spine meets the ilium of the pelvis.

The sacro-iliac joint reflex area is important in problems where the pelvis is slightly out of alignment causing problems with the lower back, the hips or the sciatic nerve, amongst others.

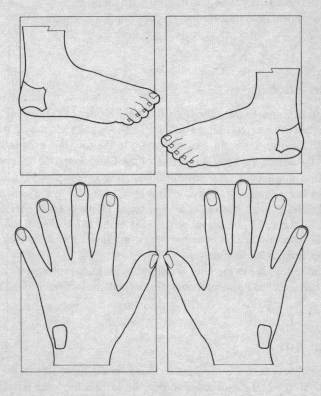

Figure 47 The reflex areas to the muscles of the pelvis

The muscles of the pelvic region

The reflex areas to the muscles of the pelvic region are in the area below the outer malleolus (ankle bone) on the lateral side of the foot, and over the base of the fifth metacarpal bone on the lateral side and top of the hand. The right foot or hand will represent the right side of the pelvis and the left foot or hand will represent the left side of the pelvis. (See figure 47).

The muscles of the pelvis refer to those muscles holding the pelvis in position. The pelvis is the large bony-shaped cavity formed by the sacrum and coccyx of the spine behind and the bones collectively called the innominate bones to the front and the sides.

The reflex areas to these muscles are important in cases of problems involving the lower spine, pelvis and hips.

The knee

The reflex area to the knee is on the outer border of the foot or hand with the left knee represented on the left foot or hand and the right knee represented on the right foot or hand. On the foot this area is found directly behind the bony projection of the fifth metatarsal bone which is often prominent on the side of the foot. The area is present in a half-moon shape extending back from this bone, half-way to the back of the heel. On the hand, the reflex area is found on the outer border of the back of the hand just below waist level of the hand. (See figure 48).

The knee joint is between the upper and lower leg and enables the lower limb to be flexible.

The reflex area to the knee is important for knee problems including arthritis, strained ligaments and problems with the cartilages of the knee.

The hip

The reflex area to the hip joint is found on the outer side of the foot or hand in a half-moon shape leading back from the knee reflex area to the back of the heel in the foot or to the wrist in the hand. The right

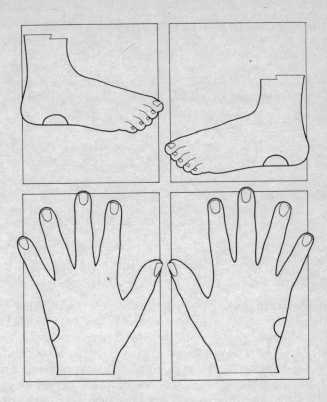

Figure 48   The reflex areas to the knees

hip is represented in the right foot or hand and the left hip is represented in the left foot or hand. (See figure 49).

The hip joint is where the femur (thigh bone) meets the pelvis.

The reflex area to the hip is important where there is a direct hip problem such as in arthritis and also with some lower back problems, pelvic problems and sciatica.

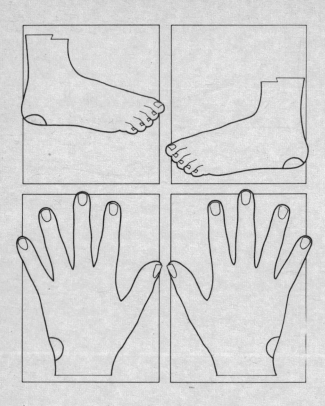

Figure 49   The reflex areas to the hips

The ovary

The reflex area to the ovary is found on the outer side of the foot or hand midway between the outer ankle bone and the back of the heel in the foot or on the outer side of the back of the hand just above the wrist. The right ovary is represented on the right foot or hand and the left ovary is represented on the left foot or hand. (See figure 50).

In the female, there are two ovaries situated one on each side in the pelvis in approximately zone three of the body. Each ovary is about the size and shape of a shelled almond. The ovaries are part of the female

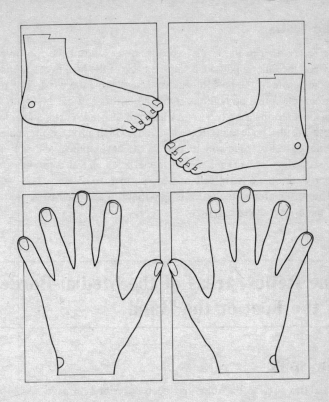

Figure 50 The reflex areas to the ovaries/testes

reproductive system and from after puberty until the menopause, they produce the female germ cells known as ova. The ovaries produce the hormones oestrogen and progesterone which influence the cyclical changes which take place during the production of ova and the menstrual cycle. In pregnancy, the normal ovarian cycle ceases.

The reflex area to the ovaries is important in all cases associated with the female reproductive glands including problems with the menstrual cycle, infertility, ovarian cysts and problems associated with the menopause.

The testis

The reflex area to the testis is on the outer side of the foot midway between the outer ankle bone and the back of the heel in the foot or on the outer side of the back of the hand just above the wrist. The reflex area will be found on both the right and left foot or hand. (Figure 50).

In the male, there are two testes which are suspended extra-abdominally. These are the male reproductive glands which produce the male sex hormone, testosterone which controls the development and activity of the secondary sex organs and characteristics and also produce, after puberty, the male germ cells called spermatozoa.

The reflex area to the testes is important in all cases associated with the male reproductive system.

The Reflex Areas of the Medial Border of the Foot or the Hand

The spine

The reflex area to the spine has been described on page 33.

The uterus

The reflex area to the uterus is found on the inner side of the foot midway between the inner malleolus (ankle bone) and the back of the heel or on the inner side of the back of the hand just above the wrist. There are reflex areas on both the right and the left foot or hand. It is also sometimes possible to find a reflex area to the uterus up the back of the leg for a few inches on either side of the Achilles tendon. (See figure 51).

The uterus is a pear-shaped muscular organ situated in the centre of the pelvis in the female. After puberty and up to the time of the menopause, cyclical changes take place in the cells of the uterus during the menstrual cycle and these changes are caused by the action of ovarian hormones. A further series of changes occur during pregnancy with the development of the foetus in the uterus.

The reflex area to the uterus is important in cases involving the female reproductive system including menstrual problems, menopausal problems, fibroids in the uterus, and in pregnancy.

The prostate gland

The reflex area to the prostate gland is on the inner side of the foot midway between the inner ankle bone and the back of the heel or on the inner side of the back of the hand just above the wrist. There are reflex areas on both the right and the left foot or hand. It is also sometimes

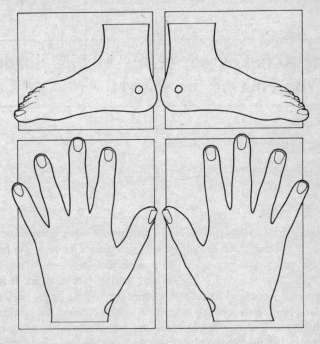

Figure 51   The reflex areas to the uterus/prostate

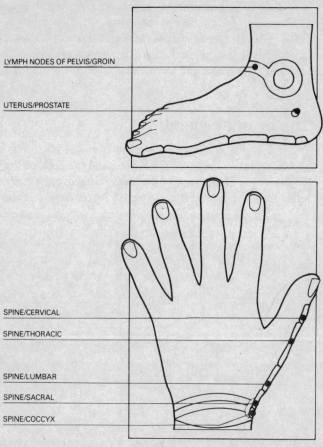

LYMPH NODES OF PELVIS/GROIN

UTERUS/PROSTATE

SPINE/CERVICAL

SPINE/THORACIC

SPINE/LUMBAR

SPINE/SACRAL

SPINE/COCCYX

*Figure 52   The reflex areas of the medial border of the feet and
the hands*

possible to find a reflex area to the prostate up the back of the leg for
a few inches on either sides of the Achilles tendon. (See figure 51).

The prostate gland is about the size and shape of a chestnut and is
situated around the neck of the bladder. Its secretion is passed into the

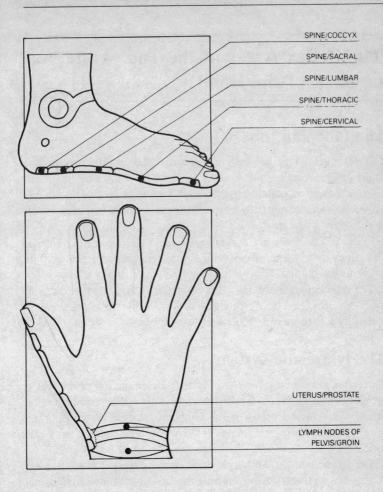

SPINE/COCCYX

SPINE/SACRAL

SPINE/LUMBAR

SPINE/THORACIC

SPINE/CERVICAL

UTERUS/PROSTATE

LYMPH NODES OF
PELVIS/GROIN

urethra and aids the transport of the spermatozoa.

The reflex area to the prostate is helpful when the prostate gland is enlarged or inflamed, with problems involving the male reproductive system and with some urinary problems such as the retention of urine.

The Reflex Areas of the Top of the Foot or Back of the Hand

The fallopian tube

The reflex area to the fallopian tube is across the top of the foot or back of the hand linking the reflex areas of the ovary and the uterus. There are reflex areas on both the right and left foot or hand. (See figure 53). This reflex area is normally massaged in conjunction with those areas to the ovary and uterus.

In the female there are two fallopian tubes and these link the right and left ovary to the uterus. The tubes act to transport the ova from the ovary to the uterus.

The reflex areas to the fallopian tubes are important when there are problems involving the reproductive system and in some cases of infertility where there is blockage of the tubes.

The lymphatic system

The reflex areas to the lymphatic system are on the top of the feet or on the back of the hands. As described for other reflex areas, the reflex areas to the various parts of the lymphatic system are in the same longitudinal and transverse zones in the foot or hand as these parts exist in the body.

The reflex areas to the lymphatic system are treated from the webs of the toes or fingers down towards the ankle bones and around each ankle bone, or towards the wrist and over the wrist bones.

The reflex areas to the upper lymph nodes are on the top of the feet or the hands just below the web between the toes or fingers. Between the big toe and second toe and between the thumb and the second finger is a reflex area for lymph drainage. The reflex area to the lymph nodes of the axilla (arm-pit) is found just below the shoulder reflex on the top of the foot or hand over the head of the fifth metatarsal or metacarpal bone. The reflex area to the breast is found across the top of the foot

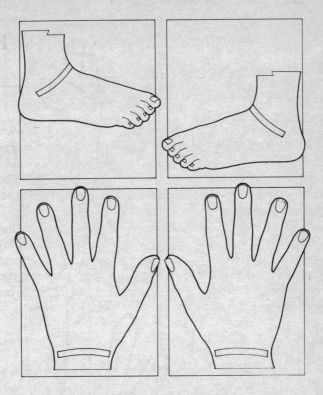

Figure 53   The reflex areas to the fallopian tubes

or hand in all five zones in the area over the metatarsal or metacarpal bones above waist level. The reflex area to the lymphatics of the abdomen is on the top of the feet or hands in all five zones. The reflex areas to the lymphatics of the pelvis and groin are in all five zones across the top of the foot between the ankle bones and around the inner and outer ankle bones, or across the back of the wrist. (See figure 55). The reflex areas are found in both the right and left feet or hands.

The lymphatic system is similar to the circulatory system in that a network of lymphatic vessels is situated throughout the body and acts to drain the tissue fluid surrounding the cells in the body. The composition

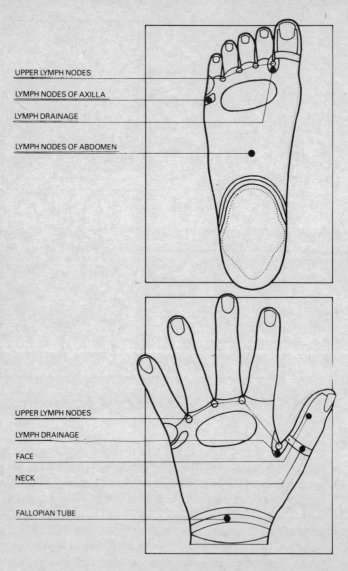

Figure 54   The reflex areas of the top of the feet and the back of the hands

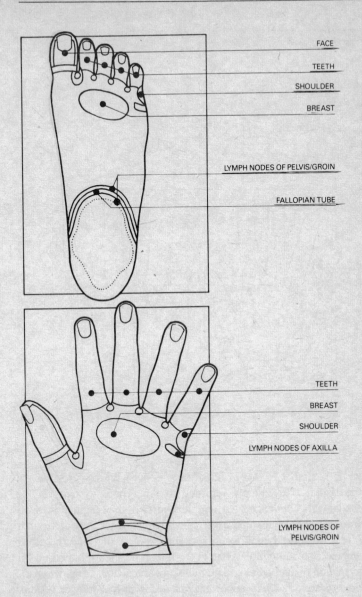

FACE

TEETH

SHOULDER

BREAST

LYMPH NODES OF PELVIS/GROIN

FALLOPIAN TUBE

TEETH

BREAST

SHOULDER

LYMPH NODES OF AXILLA

LYMPH NODES OF
PELVIS/GROIN

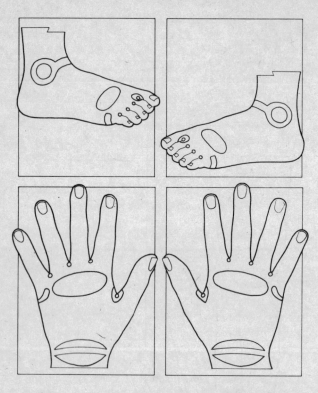

Figure 55   The reflex areas to the lymphatic system

of lymph is similar to that of blood plasma but with less protein, and all the lymph is eventually returned to the venous system via the subclavian veins in the neck. Along the course of the lymphatic vessels there are masses of lymphoid tissue called lymph nodes or lymph glands and these filter the lymph to prevent infection passing into the blood stream and also add lymphocytes to the lymph which are important for the formation of antibodies and immunological reactions. The lymphatic system is therefore a very important part of the body's defence system. The main sites of lymph nodes are in the neck, armpit, breast, abdomen,

Kirlian photographs of hands and feet, before and after treatment

Hands before treatment

Hands after treatment

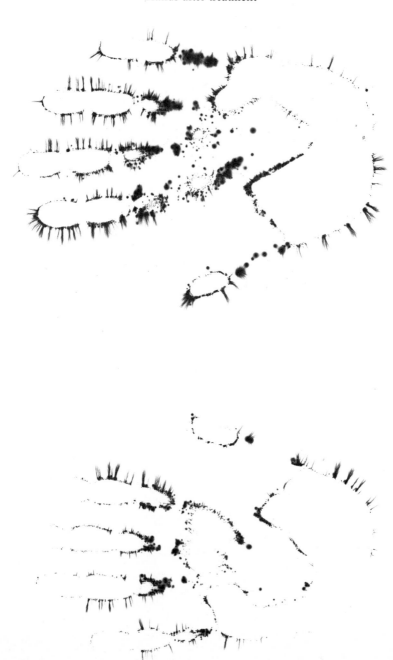

Left foot before and after treatment

Right foot before and after treatment

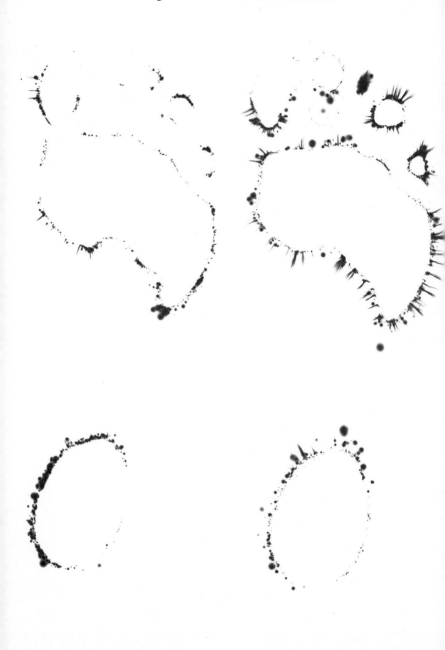

groin, pelvis and behind the knee. These nodes act to localize any infection and can become swollen in certain disorders.

The reflex areas to the lymphatic system will be important when there is infection present in the body and those lymph nodes most local to the site of the infection will be particularly involved and their reflex areas particularly important.

The skin

The reflex areas relating to the skin are in the feet or the hands in the same zones as the areas of skin to be treated are found in the body. Since the skin covers all the areas of the body, reflex areas to the skin are found in all the areas of the feet or hands.

The skin acts as a barrier against bacteria entering the body and is also involved in regulating the body temperature. The skin also contains many special nerve endings associated with the sensations of touch, pressure, pain, warmth and cold.

The reflex areas to the skin are important with any condition involving the skin such as eczema, dermatitis, rashes and psoriasis.

Order of Treatment

All the main reflex areas found in the feet and the hands have now been described but it must be remembered that every part of the foot or hand corresponds to a part of the body so every part must be massaged in a treatment session. For quick reference, the suggested order of treatment will now be summarized. (See also figures 56, 57, 58 and 59).

Right foot or right hand

Transverse zone 1 : the pituitary gland, the head and the brain, the spine, the face, the sinuses, the eye, the eustachian tube, the ear, the teeth, the shoulder and the shoulder girdle, the upper arm and the elbow, the thyroid gland, the parathyroid glands.

Transverse zone 2 : the lung, the sternum, the ribs, the diaphragm, the solar plexus, the thymus, the liver, the gall bladder, the pancreas, the stomach.

Transverse zone 3 : the small intestine, the large intestine (the ileo-caecal valve, the appendix, the ascending colon, the transverse colon), the bladder, the ureter tube, the kidney, the adrenal gland, the sciatic loop.

The lateral side of the foot or hand : the sacro-iliac joint, the muscles of the pelvis, the knee, the hip, the ovary or testis.

The medial side of the foot or hand : the uterus or the prostate gland.

The top of the foot or the back of the hand : the fallopian tube, the lymphatic system.

Left foot or left hand

Transverse zone 1 : the pituitary gland, the head and the brain, the spine, the face, the sinuses, the eye, the eustachian tube, the ear, the teeth, the shoulder and the shoulder girdle, the upper arm and the elbow, the thyroid gland, the parathyroid glands.

Transverse zone 2 : the lung, the sternum, the ribs, the heart, the diaphragm, the solar plexus, the thymus, the spleen, the pancreas, the stomach.

Transverse zone 3 : the small intestine, the large intestine (the transverse colon, the descending colon, the sigmoid colon, the rectum), the bladder, the ureter tube, the kidney, the adrenal gland, the sciatic loop.

The lateral side of the foot or hand : the sacro-iliac joint, the muscles of the pelvis, the knee, the hip, the ovary or the testis.

The medial side of the foot or hand : the uterus or the prostate gland.

The top of the foot or back of the hand : the fallopian tube, the lymphatic system.

Some of the above mentioned are slightly out of the zone mentioned but are treated alongside the areas of that zone for convenience.

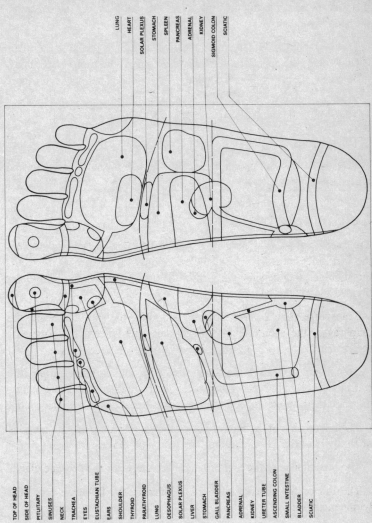

LUNG
HEART
SOLAR PLEXUS
STOMACH
SPLEEN
PANCREAS
ADRENAL
KIDNEY
SIGMOID COLON
SCIATIC

TOP OF HEAD
SIDE OF HEAD
PITUITARY
SINUSES
NECK
TRACHEA
EYES
EUSTACHIAN TUBE
EARS
SHOULDER
THYROID
PARATHYROID
LUNG
OESOPHAGUS
SOLAR PLEXUS
LIVER
STOMACH
GALL BLADDER
PANCREAS
ADRENAL
KIDNEY
URETER TUBE
ASCENDING COLON
SMALL INTESTINE
BLADDER
SCIATIC

Figure 56 The Foot Chart – the soles of the feet

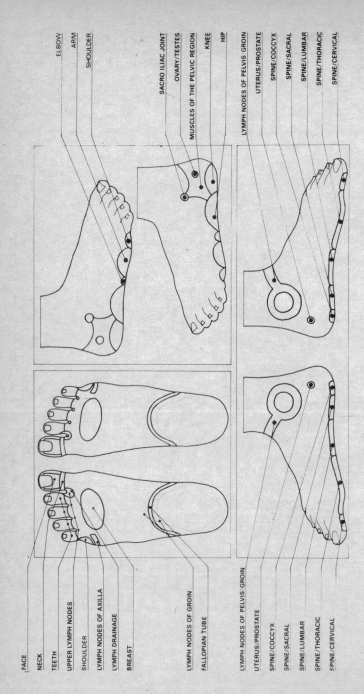

FACE
NECK
TEETH
UPPER LYMPH NODES
SHOULDER
LYMPH NODES OF AXILLA
LYMPH DRAINAGE
BREAST

LYMPH NODES OF GROIN
FALLOPIAN TUBE

LYMPH NODES OF PELVIS GROIN
UTERUS/PROSTATE
SPINE/COCCYX
SPINE/SACRAL
SPINE/LUMBAR
SPINE/THORACIC
SPINE/CERVICAL

ELBOW
ARM
SHOULDER

SACRO ILIAC JOINT
OVARY/TESTES
MUSCLES OF THE PELVIC REGION
KNEE
HIP

LYMPH NODES OF PELVIS GROIN
UTERUS/PROSTATE
SPINE/COCCYX
SPINE/SACRAL
SPINE/LUMBAR
SPINE/THORACIC
SPINE/CERVICAL

Figure 57   The Foot Chart – the tops and sides of the feet

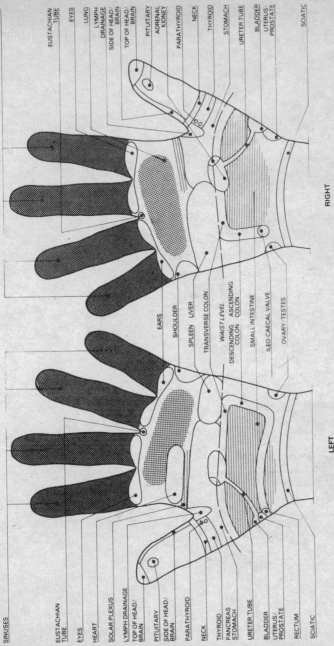

SINUSES

EUSTACHIAN
TUBE

EYES

HEART

SOLAR PLEXUS

LYMPH DRAINAGE

TOP OF HEAD/
BRAIN

PITUITARY

SIDE OF HEAD/
BRAIN

PARATHYROID

NECK

THYROID

PANCREAS
STOMACH

URETER TUBE

BLADDER

UTERUS/
PROSTATE

RECTUM

SCIATIC

LEFT

EARS

SHOULDER

SPLEEN   LIVER

TRANSVERSE COLON

WAIST LEVEL

DESCENDING   ASCENDING
COLON   COLON

SMALL INTESTINE

ILEO-CAECAL VALVE

OVARY TESTES

RIGHT

SINUSES

EUSTACHIAN
TUBE

EYES

LUNG

LYMPH
DRAINAGE

SIDE OF HEAD/
BRAIN

TOP OF HEAD/
BRAIN

PITUITARY

ADRENAL
KIDNEY

PARATHYROID

NECK

THYROID

STOMACH

URETER TUBE

BLADDER

UTERUS/
PROSTATE

SCIATIC

Figure 58   The Hand Chart — the palms of the hands

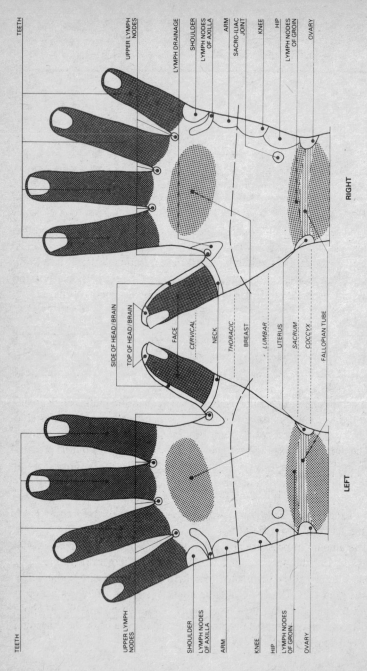

Figure 59 The Hand Chart – the backs of the hands

3 How Reflexology Treatment is Given – The Massage Technique

Having seen where all the reflex areas are positioned in the feet and the hands, we will look at how these areas will be treated. There are various different methods of treatment. The different training schools may well teach different applications of the method and none are particularly right or wrong – the overall importance is to achieve good results.

The Basic Technique

In most instances, the thumb is used to apply pressure to the reflex areas. The right or left thumb can be used – whichever is most comfortable – and a skilled practitioner will become adept at using either thumb.

The thumb will be held bent, and the side and end of the thumb pressed onto the part of the foot or hand to be treated. The other fingers of the hand will rest gently round the foot or hand, and the other hand will be used to support the area being worked on so will be placed on the top of the foot or hand when working on the sole of the foot or palm of the hand. (See figure 60).

The amount of pressure applied to the reflex area will depend on the sensitivity of the person being worked on. Dr Fitzgerald, in his early Zone Therapy work, estimated it as between two and ten pounds. The lower limit seems more acceptable nowadays and it is always better to work too gently rather than too heavily. It should be possible to apply sufficient pressure without the practitioner feeling that he or she is needing to exert much effort.

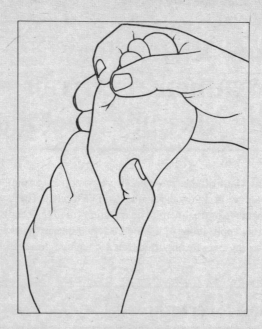

Figure 60   The angle of the thumb for treatment

To move on to the next reflex point, the thumb is moved off the reflex area by easing back slightly and then easing forward onto the next area. The thumb will be kept bent and also kept in contact with the foot or hand. (See figure 61).

Each movement should be a definite one and the thumb should not rub over the skin. Remember that each reflex area is only about the size of a pin's head so a very precise action is required to locate the reflex areas exactly.

In order not to insert the nail into the skin when giving the treatment – apart from having short nails – the practitioner presses very slightly back on each point rather than pressing in forward.

On some areas of the feet or hands it is easier to apply the massage with a finger rather than the thumb. The same technique will, however, be employed using the side and end of the finger to press onto the reflex

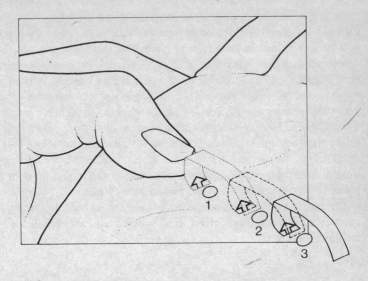

*Figure 61   The movement of the thumb for treatment.   The space
between points 1, 2 and 3 is exaggerated in order to show the
movement pattern. In practice, the points are adjacent to each other*

area. The fingers are sometimes more convenient when working on the
side of the foot for areas such as the shoulder reflex and the reproductive
gland reflexes.

Where possible, working from one reflex area to another is in a forward
direction meaning that the tip of the thumb or finger is pointing in the
direction in which one is working.

To stay on the same reflex point

If extra massage is required to an area, then the technique described above
can be adapted. The thumb will be pressed onto an area and then eased
off slightly in a backward direction and then pressure applied again. This
will produce a circular type movement but the thumb will not actually
circle round on the skin but rather in the way in which the pressure is
applied, released and reapplied.

At first it may seem difficult to keep the thumb bent nearly all the time but with practise this method becomes much easier and the hands will be able to remain in a relaxed manner as treatment is given.

Another technique often described involves applying pressure with a bent thumb, then straightening the thumb and then bending it again to move across the reflex areas. This method is not recommended since it is very wearing on the thumb joints, though it can achieve results. Yet another technique involves circling around quite definitely on each reflex point and again, although this may achieve results, it is a much more tiring exercise and does not feel so pleasant to the person being treated. Similarly, if a prodding action is used on each point, the overall effect is not very pleasant to the person being treated.

The massage movements on the feet or hand should be slow and gentle in order to have a relaxing effect. Harsh, quick movements will not be comfortable.

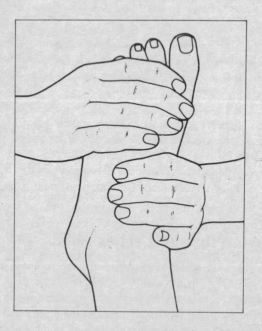

Figure 62   'Wringing' the foot

At the end of a treatment session, when all the reflex areas have been massaged, the practitioner will normally finish with some general massage movements on the feet or hands. These may include a wringing action on the feet with the hands placed around the opposite sides of the foot or hand and the hands 'wrung' apart — this action has a beneficial effect on the general structure of the foot by 'spreading' the bones out. It can also be seen as 'spreading' the organs of the body out and in particular the lung area which is found over the metatarsal or metacarpal bones to which this movement is particularly applied. (See figure 62).

Another action used is to 'knead' the foot or hand by placing the flat portion of the clenched hand formed by the proximal phalanges onto the arch of the foot with the other hand flat on top of the foot — both hands are then pressed onto the foot and circled round in a 'kneading' manner and this again helps the general structure of the foot. (See figure 63). A similar action can be carried out on the hand.

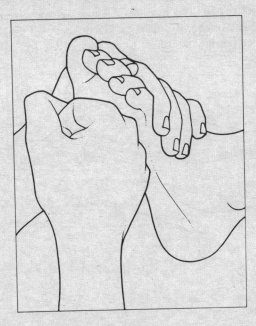

Figure 63   'Kneading' the foot

A stroking action on the top of the feet or backs of the hands can help the circulation to these areas and stimulate the lymphatic circulation. It is also helpful if there is swelling of the foot or hand. This action begins at the roots of the toes or fingers with the fingers stroking down the foot or hand followed by a similar action by the pad of the wrist. (Figure 64).

An additional very beneficial movement involves rotation of each toe or finger in turn − rotating in both a clockwise and anti-clockwise direction with the other hand supporting the joint being rotated. (Figure 65).

Rotating the big toes or thumbs is similar to rotating the neck and if the neck is very stiff these joints will be found to be very stiff. Rotation of the ankles also aids the suppleness of the foot and encourages a better blood circulation to the foot. Likewise for the rotation of the wrists.

Often people are somewhat apprehensive about having their feet touched but pleasant massage techniques should soon overcome these worries. Any fear that the treatment may tickle is also unnecessary since in the majority of cases a firm, definite massage movement is used. At the onset of a treatment session, a practitioner will massage the feet generally, to enable the patient to get used to the feet being touched.

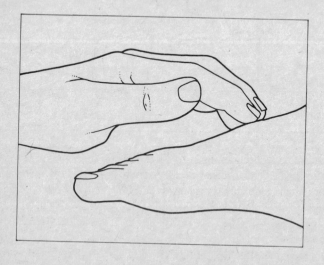

Figure 64   Massage to the top of the foot

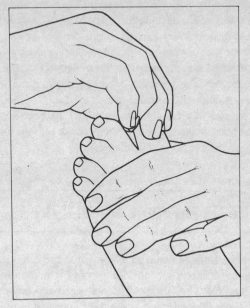

Figure 65   Rotation of the big toe

Gadgets

Beware of gadgets claiming to give Reflexology treatment. The various types of sandals and insoles with raised, nobbled surfaces which are said to work on the reflex areas may have some effect but this effect is random and there is the risk of over-stimulating certain areas whilst leaving other areas untreated. In fact to many, these items inflict considerable discomfort to the feet.

Foot and hand rollers, similar in shape to rolling-pins, but with corrugated edges can be used to roll the sole of the foot over or can be rolled between the palms of the hands. These again, are probably not precise enough to give a thorough treatment but they can be beneficial in relaxing the feet or hands and thereby relaxing the whole body. The rollers are also helpful when circulation in the feet or hands is poor, and also to improve the muscle tone of the feet and hands.

However, there is no better substitute for giving Reflexology treatment than to give the massage by hand. By understanding the method and knowing the positions of the reflex areas, the trained practitioner will be able to treat the whole body, and to adjust the pressure applied to suit the person being treated. The whole experience of Reflexology should therefore be one of pleasure and relaxation.

What the Treatment Feels Like

When the precise form of massage is applied to the reflex areas in the feet or the hands, different feelings will be present in the various areas. Some areas may feel very sharp when massaged and often the patient thinks that the practitioner is just using the finger nail to press into the foot. Others describe this sharpness as being like a thorn or piece of glass pressing into the foot. When some areas are massaged a duller pain is felt, rather as if the area is bruised. In other areas, just the sensation of a firm pressure will be felt.

The different tendernesses felt in the different reflex areas indicate to the practitioner which parts of the body are not working well and which are. The more tender the reflex area, the more out of balance the corresponding part of the body is.

With each individual, the sensitivity of the feet or hands will differ and some people may show many tender reflex areas but be in reasonably good health whilst others may show less tender reflex areas but be in poor health. The different sensitivities of the reflex areas will be interpreted in accordance with the overall sensitivity of the feet or hands. Even in the same individual, the sensitivity of the feet or hands can vary from one treatment session to another depending on factors such as the time of day of the treatment, the type of mood the person is in and of course their state of health on that occasion. Sometimes, when people first experience Reflexology treatment, the reflex areas appear very insensitive even though the person is not in good health. In these cases feet usually become more sensitive after the second or third treatment sessions as the energy flow to the feet improves. For often people rarely think of their feet unless they cause some problem and they need to increase their awareness of the feet before the reflex areas begin to respond sensitively to the treatment. The reflex areas in the hands are usually less sensitive than those in the feet, though as Reflexology massage is carried out on the hands, the reflex areas do become more sensitive. It appears, however, that the treatment still works even if tender areas are not felt in the feet or hands, and this is one of the reasons why it is important to understand which reflex areas are important in different conditions.

In most cases the reflex areas to those parts of the body out of balance appear to be tender and as treatment progresses and the patient responds, the reflex areas become less sensitive. The ideal is that no tender reflex areas are found in the feet representing total balance throughout the body. This state rarely occurs though, since most people will experience some slight tension or weakness in the body and the treatment, being extremely sensitive, will identify this through the tender areas in the feet or hands.

The tender areas described will only be felt when the reflex area is massaged in the precise way. These tendernesses will not be experienced when walking barefoot but should the foot be placed firmly on an object such as a stone or piece of gravel, it might well be that the pain felt would be exaggerated if the stone had pressed on a reflex area which represented a part of the body which was out of balance. A similar effect would occur with the hands if an object was pressed firmly into the hands and touched a reflex area corresponding to a part of the body which was out of balance.

The treatment should never be extremely uncomfortable since the practitioner will adjust the amount of pressure applied to suit the individual. If there is great sensitivity in the reflex areas, then a lighter pressure should be applied. Particular care is needed when the feet are arthritic, and this is one instance where there might be slightly more discomfort in the feet following treatment — but only for a short while. In general, following a treatment session, the feet should feel most comfortable and often patients may say that their feet feel 'tingly' and light, or that it feels as if they are 'walking on air'.

4 Foot and Hand Care

Having seen how in the feet and the hands, every part of these areas represents a part of the body, the great importance of the feet and hands must be obvious. In general, people tend to take better care of their hands than their feet, probably because they are more on view to themselves and others, and anything wrong with them is more noticeably seen or felt. The feet, being protected for most of the time in socks, stockings and shoes are often rather neglected, and attention is only paid to them if for some one reason they are painful or ache. It is possible that problems with the feet or hands can relate to problems in the underlying reflex areas though it is not possible to say whether the foot or hand problem causes the problem in the body or if the foot or hand problem arises due to a problem in the body. This point should, however, be remembered and better care of the feet and hands encouraged.

Regular washing should be followed by careful drying to prevent cracks developing and if areas become hardened a hand or foot cream should be massaged into the hands or feet. Problems such as corns, verrucas and athlete's foot should all be dealt with and a chiropodist consulted for persistent problems.

Everything about the feet or hands will be important to the Reflexology practitioner. Since treatment is normally given to the feet these will be considered in more detail. When a patient is seated with shoes and socks removed the practitioner will study the feet noting the temperature, skin condition, muscle tone, tissue structure and bone structure.

The temperature of the feet or hands will be significant. If the feet or hands are very cold then poor blood circulation is indicated and this may also suggest that other areas of the body may receive a poor blood circulation. Where the blood circulation to the feet or hands or both is poor, it is important that the person wears warm socks and gloves in

the cold weather − an obvious point but often overlooked. If the feet
or hands perspire a lot then this may indicate a glandular imbalance in
the body. In these conditions, it is better for the person to wear socks,
shoes, gloves in natural fibres rather than synthetic fibres which may
accentuate the problem.

The skin condition of the feet and hands may also relate to glandular
problems especially if they are excessively dry. In addition, areas of hard
skin on the feet usually form due to extra pressure being placed on either
areas and may be related to a postural imbalance in the body. Wearing
high-heeled shoes can create this type of problem. Poor circulation in
the feet or hands may also lead to dryness of the skin. If an area of the
foot is infected such as by a verruca or athlete's foot then this part of
the foot will not be treated but the corresponding reflex area in the hand
will be treated instead. Similarly, if there are blisters or varicose veins,
these areas will be left alone. It may well be that where there are verrucas,
athlete's foot or corns, this may relate to a problem in the underlying
reflex area. For example, a corn between the second and third toes may
indicate an eye problem; a verruca on the top of the pad of the big toe
may indicate a head problem such as headaches or migraine.

The muscle tone of the foot may relate to the muscle tone throughout
the whole body. If the feet feel rather 'flabby' then there may be poor
muscle tone in the body, and if the flabbiness is only in certain areas
then this may directly relate to the part of the body to which this part
of the foot corresponds. Similarly, if the muscles of the feet feel very
tight, this may relate to tension in the body or in the areas represented
by the parts of the foot which are tight.

The tissue structure of the foot may relate to the tissue structure of
the body and if there is swelling of the foot, there may be swelling in
the corresponding part of the body. For example, swelling around the
ankles may indicate swelling in the pelvis, i.e. congestion in the pelvis.
Swelling of the ankles can, however, also relate to problems with
the lymphatic system, kidneys, heart or circulation. If the swelling
is around the base of the toes, then this may indicate congestion in
the upper thorax.

The bony structure of the foot can also indicate problems in the body.
A bunion, which is an enlargement of the head of the first metatarsal
bone where it articulates with the big toe, may relate to a problem with

the neck, cervical spine or thyroid. Bunions often develop in women who wear shoes which are too narrow for the foot, and apart from the discomfort to the foot and the problem then of finding comfortable shoes, bunions may also cause trouble in other parts of the body. Hammer toes may relate to problems involving the head areas including the sinuses and the teeth. Ingrowing toe-nails by pressing on the reflex area to the top of the head may cause headaches. Flat feet and fallen arches may affect the reflex areas to the spine and a flattened transverse arch may affect the shoulder girdle and thoracic organs such as the lungs and heart. If the cuneiform bones are sunken this may affect the small intestines and if there is injury around the inner or outer ankle bones, this may affect the pelvis or the hips. Damage to the top of the foot in the region of the reflex area to the breast may affect the breast tissue such as by the formation of lumps.

All of the examples mentioned can equally well be applied to the hands and when you start to consider the feet and hands in terms of the reflex areas they become even more important than you previously imagined. The need to take great care of the feet and hands is very evident.

5 How the Treatment Works

As yet it is not clear exactly what happens when the reflex areas in the hands or the feet are massaged to bring about an effect in a distant part of the body. No doubt in future years this will be explained and this will certainly contribute to making Reflexology a more acceptable form of treatment to those who feel that there has to be a 'scientific' explanation for something before it can possibly be considered effective.

As you now know, Reflexology works on a system of energy zones which act longitudinally throughout the body ending in the feet and the hands. By working on the reflex areas in the hands and the feet, it is possible to detect imbalances in these energy zones and to correct the flow of energy within the zone and thus right the condition present.

When the reflex areas are worked on there is an increase in the blood circulation to the corresponding part of the body and this is beneficial since it is through the blood circulation that the various parts of the body receive their supply of nutrients, and the blood also carries away from the areas waste products which can then be removed from the body through one of the eliminating systems. Also, by working on the reflex areas it is possible to reduce the nerve tension present in the corresponding parts of the body and this is another important factor since it is generally accepted that at least 60 to 70 percent of all disorders are due to nerve tension.

In some areas of the feet or hands, it may be possible for the practitioner to feel the presence of crystal deposits which will represent an imbalance in the corresponding part of the body. By massaging these crystals, it is possible to cause them to be broken down and taken up by the blood circulation to be eliminated from the body. It is sometimes stated that the whole purpose of the Reflexology massage is to search out these crystals in the feet or hands and disperse them but this is not the sole purpose of the method and the crystals will not always be found even though a reflex area appears to be tender.

Another effect of the treatment is on the healing forces which exist in the body. With many complaints, provided that they are not too serious, the body has the ability to put itself right by the action of its healing forces present. By giving Reflexology treatment, the self-healing properties of the body are stimulated to encourage and hasten repair and improvement. In many ways, Reflexology can be considered as one of the most natural of the natural therapies since it acts to encourage and assist the body to put itself right without involving any other factors.

Diagnosis

Through the massage of all the reflex areas of the feet or the hands, the whole body can be treated and brought back into balance, and the treatment can therefore be used to treat a great number of different disorders some of which will be mentioned later. The method can also be used for diagnosis since, by finding which reflex areas are tender, the practitioner is alerted to which parts of the body are out of balance. This diagnostic aspect is sometimes used by pracititioners in other natural medicine fields who then use their own therapies to treat the condition. It must be remembered that the diagnosis is of the parts of the body which are out of balance and not of specific, named disorders.

Preventative Treatment

There is a growing awareness of people nowadays that they should take a greater responsibility for their own health and, rather than waiting until they become ill and then seeking treatment, try and prevent illness from occurring. One of the main areas in which this has been encouraged has been through a healthy diet. Natural therapies such as Reflexology can also be used to maintain good health. By having regular treatment sessions at monthly or two-monthly intervals, the state of the functioning of the body can be diagnosed and if, by the appearance of tender reflex areas, problems are indicated, these can then be treated before they have shown as any serious symptoms. The treatment is also extremely relaxing and for this reason is of great benefit to everyone. By enabling the body to relax, self-healing functions are more readily carried out to enable the smooth functioning of the whole body.

Reactions to Treatment

One of the most common reasons which patients will give for seeking the help of an 'alternative' therapy is that they are worried about the possible side-effects which conventional drug treatment can often cause. These unpleasant side effects can be avoided by trying a natural therapy, though one must not totally discount the value of certain traditional medicine methods which can in certain cases be life-saving.

As with all natural therapies, it is sometimes possible that as a result of Reflexology treatment some form of healing reaction may occur as the body tries to rid itself of unwanted toxic material. The type of reaction that occurs will depend on the system or systems of the body which are congested but in the hands of a skilled practitioner these reactions should not be too severe. Remember that in many cases symptoms have been building up over a period of time and it may take a little time to clear the condition. If there are many toxins present in the system it would be unwise to try and clear them too fast which might put a great strain on an already imbalanced body.

These healing reactions are cleansing reactions and will therefore appear as increased activity of the eliminating systems of the body. One of the most common reactions to treatment is that the kidneys and urinary system are stimulated and the need to pass water is more frequent. If the digestive system is at fault, a person may feel slightly nauseous after treatment or may find increased activity of the bowels. Digestive 'noises' may also increase during and after treatment. If someone suffers from catarrh or sinus congestion, then symptoms similar to those of a cold may appear after treatment, with the nose and eyes running as the congestion is cleared. Where the respiratory system is at fault, the patient may cough more after treatment with the clearing of mucus. With skin problems, there may be a flare up of a rash — this is particularly so if the skin problem has been treated previously with suppressive ointments and creams. Other reactions to the treatment may include different sleeping patterns: either deeper sleep or sometimes more disturbed sleep with more vivid recollection of dreams. Emotional differences may also occur and depression with weeping may result from treatment as the toxins clear from the system and the emotions 'unwind'. It is also possible that symptoms present in the past but no longer apparent, may be re-established as the body tries to clear the problem totally. With joint problems and in particular arthritic conditions, there may be a slight increase in the pain felt following treatment.

These reactions to treatment should certainly not put people off treatment as they may not necessarily occur and, as mentioned before, if treatment is given correctly the degree of reaction can be controlled.

After treatment the patient should feel very relaxed and, often, tired which is the body's way of telling the person to rest for the maximum benefit. In others, there may be an increased feeling of energy and also a feeling of well-being. Patients may feel warm after treatment due to the improved blood supply while others may feel rather shivery as the body's energy is directed inwards for healing.

Whatever the reactions that occur, they should pass off in a few hours or days as the body becomes freer of toxins, less tense and more in balance resulting in better health.

Kirlian Photography

This method can be used to show that a Reflexology treatment is able to affect the energy fields in the body. Kirlian Photography was first described by a Russian husband and wife, Semyon and Valentia Kirlian. To take a Kirlain photograph, the hands or feet are placed on a piece of photo paper on top of the Kirlian machine and the machine gives out a high-frequency field. The energy surrounding the hands or the feet repels this field and this causes a pattern of interference which is photographed. If there is a deficiency of the energy body around the hands or feet, then the energy from the machine goes into space without meeting a resistance and no picture is produced.

In general, the hands reflect the psychological aspects of the person and the feet reflect the medical aspects of the person. The areas photographed can also be interpreted in relation to the reflex areas found in the hands and the feet. The illustrations between pages 96-97 show the different pictures achieved before and after a Reflexology treatment.

For the hands, there is a marked increase in the energy fields following treatment. For the feet, the difference is not so obvious though it must be noted that it does appear to be more difficult to take good photographs of the feet with this method. A detailed interpretation of the photographs will not be given here but one of the most interesting points to show is the presence of toxins in certain areas which are shown as small black dots. In the feet, after treatment, less toxins were evident in the areas corresponding to the neck, cervical spine, the sinuses, the lungs, the liver, the thyroid and the pelvic areas. There was, however, an increase in the toxins showing in the spleen. In the hands, after treatment, again less toxins were evident in the areas corresponding to the neck and cervical spine. The sinuses and lungs, however, showed the presence of more toxins. The patient in question had just developed a heavy cold and bad cough and the areas indicating the presence of toxins related to these conditions. The fact that toxins were more evident, after treatment, in the hands in the sinuses and lung areas may suggest that the toxins had been stimulated to be dispersed but obviously the effect of the treatment is not instantaneous. The patient did report that the afternoon following the treatment, she coughed extensively and also perspired heavily which was unusual for her but both of these factors indicate that the body was ridding itself of toxins. Also in the hands after treatment, there was a more balanced and definite energy pattern indicating that the treatment had also helped on the psychological level.

Kirlian photography offers an interesting means of seeing the effect of Reflexology treatment and much can be diagnosed about the physical and mental aspects of the patient from these photographs.

6 The Treatment Session

Reflexology treatment nowadays is quite widely available and at most natural therapy centres there will be a practising Reflexologist. Most practitioners are in private practice and their addresses can be obtained from the appropriate representative bodies (see page 180). It is not unusual to find practitioners working from home since a relatively small space is required as a treatment room and few extra fixtures and fittings.

The ideal treatment chair is a recliner chair which will allow the patient to sit in a comfortable position with feet raised to a height which is comfortable for the practitioner to work on. This type of chair will support the back but enable the patient to be in a sitting position in which they can face the practitioner. This position will also mean that the leg is bent slightly at the groin and the knee will be bent. With the knee bent and from knee to ankle totally supported, the feet are in their most relaxed position. If the knee is not bent and the leg therefore straight, the foot will be slightly tense.

A treatment session will last for about one hour and this will include the time taken to settle the patient in the treatment chair with shoes and socks removed and for these items to be put on again after treatment. There is no need for any further undressing as only the feet (or hands) will be treated. The actual length of the treatment will thus be about three-quarters of an hour and in this time all the reflex areas of both feet will be treated. If treatment is given to the hands instead of the feet, then the treatment time is slightly shorter since the areas to be massaged are not as large. For children, the length of a treatment session may also be slightly shorter since again the feet are smaller. Moreover, it is probably unlikely that a child will sit quietly for as long a period.

For most conditions, a course of treatment will be required and each treatment is usually given at weekly or sometimes twice weekly intervals. Treatment is not normally given more frequently than this since it is possible to overtreat. As a very general guide, a course of about six to eight treatments will be required but it should be stressed that this is only a guide. For serious conditions, many more treatments may be necessary and for minor problems fewer treatments may be required. The treatment is never likely to be once only though, and with all conditions it is sensible to expect to have to have a minimum of three to four treatments. The reason for this is that although one or two treatments may seem to have produced good results, it is important to balance up the whole body to ensure that the problem does not return in a short space of time.

Although weekly treatments are recommended, it may be that, as the condition responds, the interval between treatments can be extended. Many people sensibly continue with treatment at intervals of, for example, one, two or three months having had a condition corrected, as they are keen to maintain their improved state of health and see that the treatment may prevent other problems from occurring.

Once people have experienced a course of treatment, it is usually found that if another symptom occurs or the same symptoms for which they had been treated reoccur, then a short refresher course of treatment is all that is needed. It does seem that once people have been treated successfully by the method, on future occasions they seem to respond to the method more quickly. The fact that a treatment session lasts for about one hour is sometimes offputting to patients but these are the people who probably most need to sit down and relax for an hour.

Often patients will express surprise at how quickly the treatment hour passes. The mere fact of sitting and doing nothing for an hour is of tremendous value to most people since nowadays many people lead such busy, stressful lives.

As will be seen in the next chapter, Reflexology treatment can be used to treat a wide range of disorders so it is more than likely that if a person decides to try the method, it will help in some way. There are certain cases, however, when treatment would not be given or where extra care is required when giving the treatment and these cases will include such disorders as thrombosis, phlebitis, certain heart disorders, osteoporosis, arthritis in the feet, diabetes and pregnancy. Of these, it may be possible for treatment to be given and the trained practitioner would be able to give suitable advice.

Self-treatment

It is possible to use Reflexology for self-treatment and often the hands are more suitable for self-treatment since they are more readily accessible. The feet can be worked on but not in a particularly relaxed position. The use of self-treatment for minor conditions may often be successful but for more serious conditions it is important that the person fully understands how to give the treatment. Sometimes, a practitioner will recommend to a patient that they work on certain reflex areas on their hands or feet in between their treatment sessions and this will apply more often to those reflex areas which are more easily located such as the head reflex area (for headaches, migraines), the sinus reflex areas (for catarrh and blocked sinuses), the spine reflex area (for backache), the neck reflex area (for a stiff neck) and the solar plexus reflex area (to release tension).

It is important to remember that it is possible to overwork the reflex areas which might upset the balance in the body, probably temporarily, but with possible unpleasant effects. For this reason, self-treatment should only be used as indicated by a practitioner or with a sound understanding of what the method is doing.

7 The Treatment of Different Disorders

It must be remembered that with any condition, all the reflex areas in the feet or hands will be massaged in order to try and balance up all the systems in the body and therefore correct not only the symptoms which are present but also the cause of the symptoms. It will, however, be obvious that in certain conditions, certain reflex areas will be of greater importance either because they are directly involved in the condition or are involved in the possible cause of the condition. In many cases, there may well be several different complaints, some of which may often be connected. By being able to treat the whole body through the feet or the hands, all of the different complaints can be treated by the one method.

One hundred different examples of disorders will now be looked at and with each of these the important reflex areas will be mentioned. These will include the reflex areas which are directly related to the condition (DR) and the reflex areas which may be associated with the condition (AR), though with the latter group not all of these areas may be of importance for every individual with the condition.

As a guide to the different examples given they will first be listed under the system of the body to which they mainly relate, as follows:

The head – Bell's palsy, catarrh, coma, conjunctivitis, deafness, depression, earache, epilepsy, eye strain, glaucoma, hay fever, headaches, insomnia, Ménière's disease, meningitis, migraine, neuralgia, rhinitis, sinusitis, stroke, tear ducts blocked, tinnitus, toothache, vertigo.

The musculo-skeletal system – arthritis, backache, bursitis, cramp, fibrositis, foot problems, fractures, frozen shoulder, gout, knee pains, lumbago, multiple sclerosis, muscle strains, neck stiffness, paralysis, Parkinson's disease, rheumatism, sciatica, spondylitis, tennis elbow, tenosynovitis.

The endocrine system − diabetes, fibroids, goitre, hypoglycaemia, infertility, menopause, menstrual problems, ovarian cyst, pregnancy, pre-menstrual tension, tension, thyroid imbalance.

The respiratory system − asthma, bronchitis, cough, emphysema, pleurisy.

The heart and the circulatory system − angina, chilblains, heart attack, hypertension, hypotension, phlebitis, Raynaud's disease, thrombosis, varicose veins.

The lymphatic system − breast cysts, cancer, infection, mastitis, tonsilitis.

The digestive system − allergies, anorexia, colitis, constipation, diarrhoea, diverticulitis, flatulence, gall stones, haemorrhoids, hepatitis, hernia, indigestion, jaundice, ulcers.

The urinary system − cystitis, incontinence, kidney stones, nephritis, prostate gland enlargement.

The skin − acne, dermatitis, eczema, psoriasis, shingles.

One Hundred Disorders

1 Acne

This is a skin disorder often affecting adolescents where spots appear on the face, neck, back and chest. It can be due to hormonal imbalances and dietary factors and often causes stress to the person affected because of their appearance.

DR: zones relating to skin affected, i.e. face, neck, back, chest.
AR: pituitary, thyroid, adrenals, reproductive areas, digestive areas, liver, solar plexus, kidneys, upper lymphatic areas.

2 Allergies

An allergy is a hyper-sensitivity of a part of the body to a substance and the most common allergies involve food allergies causing digestive upsets, headaches and skin rashes, contact allergies affecting the skin and chemical allergies affecting any of the body systems such as the digestive, respiratory, urinary and skin. The treatment will help to make the body less sensitive to the offending substances but avoidance of these substances if known is recommended initially.

DR: those areas where allergic reaction is shown, i.e. digestive areas, skin, respiratory areas.

AR: adrenals, solar plexus, spleen.

3 Angina

This is where a severe pain is felt in the heart area of the chest, which can also sometimes spread towards the left shoulder and down the left arm. The pain is of short duration and is due to insufficient oxygen reaching the heart muscles. Persistent angina can often lead to a heart attack.

DR: heart.

AR: solar plexus, adrenals, shoulder and arm (if pain felt in these areas).

4 Anorexia

In this condition there is a loss of appetite for food and a resultant aversion to food can occur. Psychological factors are often involved.

DR: stomach.

AR: solar plexus, pituitary, thyroid, adrenals, reproductive areas.

5 Arthritis

This is where there is pain and inflammation of a joint or joints. There are many different types of arthritis but the more common forms are the following. Osteoarthritis, which is due to wear and tear in the joints and usually affects the weight-bearing joints such as the hips and knees, though also the fingers. The cartilage between the bones of the joint wears down to give rough, hard edges to the bones and the formation of 'knobbly'

areas at the joints. Or rheumatoid arthritis where the cartilage between the bones wears away and is replaced by scar tissue which makes the joint movements awkward and may pull the joint slightly out of line. Any of the joints of the body can be affected by arthritis though the most common ones affected are the spine, hip, knee, shoulder and finger joints. Depending on the severity of the disorder, treatment can help to relieve pain and inflammation and in some cases can bring about a very good improvement. **DR**: areas to joints affected, direct massage for zone related area of body e.g. elbow for knee, shoulder for hip, toes for fingers.
AR: parathyroids, adrenals, solar plexus, kidneys, pituitary. A good general treatment is also required in many cases of arthritis since it can have a lowering effect on the whole body.

6   Asthma

In this condition the lungs are affected and breathing difficulties including breathlessness, a feeling of suffocation, coughing and wheezing are experienced due to generalized narrowing of the air passageways. Allergy factors including foods, and stress may cause asthma attacks.
DR: lungs, bronchi.
AR: solar plexus, diaphragm, adrenals, heart, digestive areas, spine (cervical, thoracic areas), pituitary.

7   Backache

Many people suffer from backache either as a result of a direct injury to the back or due to a weakness in a region of the back which will flare up when under undue strain. Any region of the spine may be affected with the most common sites of pain being in the cervical and lumbar regions. The pain may be caused by muscle or ligament damage, a slipped disc or arthritis in a related area.
DR: spine, neck.
AR: adrenals, solar plexus, areas supplied by spinal nerves.

8 Bell's palsy

In this condition there is distortion of the face due to damage to the facial nerve and there may be pain, muscle weakness and tingling of the skin. One of the characteristics of the condition is the lopsided smile.
DR: face, head, brain.
AR: adrenals, solar plexus, upper spine.

9 Breast cysts

Cysts or lumps in the breast need not be serious but can cause discomfort.
DR: breast.
AR: lymphatic areas, especially axillary nodes.

10 Bronchitis

This is where there is inflammation of the bronchi, the air passageways of the lungs, with a dry cough or the coughing up of mucus and slight fever, back pain and a sore throat. Treatment can be helpful to those with a tendency to develop bronchitis, by strengthening the body's systems.
DR: bronchi, lungs, throat.
AR: lymphatic areas, spine, pituitary (if fever), adrenals, solar plexus.

11 Bursitis

A bursa is a small fluid-filled sac found between muscles, between tendon and bone and between skin and bone which allows movement without friction between these surfaces. A bursa can become inflamed and cause swelling and pain. Areas most commonly affected are the shoulder, elbow and big toe. The latter is what is called a bunion and can be caused by ill-fitting shoes.
DR: area affected, e.g. shoulder, elbow, thumb joint (as zone-related are for big toe joint is working on feet).
AR: adrenals, parathyroids, solar plexus.

12 Cancer

This general term refers to malignant growths found in the body. Any part of the body can be affected and more than one part may be involved. The treatment in the later stages of the condition may not be able to clear the condition but it can be helpful to the general physical and mental state of the person affected.

DR: areas affected.
AR: lymphatic areas, spleen.

13 Catarrh

This refers to inflammation of a mucus membrane with a constant flow of mucus and is usually used in connection with the nose where there are symptoms, similar to a cold, but which never seem to clear up. The nose can be blocked but also sometimes discharging.

DR: nose, sinuses.
AR: head, eyes, upper lymph nodes, digestive areas.

14 Chilblains

These usually affect the fingers or toes and there is swelling, redness and extreme irritation of these parts. The blood vessels of the area are unable to adjust correctly to changes in outside temperature and though more normal in winter when it is cold, they can also occur due to excessive heat.

DR: zone related area to affected part (fingers for toes or vice versa), heart.
AR: adrenals, digestive system, liver, lymphatic areas.

15 Colitis

In this condition the colon (large intestine) is inflamed resulting in abdominal pains and diarrhoea. Apart from diet, a stress factor is often involved.

DR: large intestine.
AR: small intestine, rectum, adrenals, solar plexus.

16 Coma

This is a complete loss of consciousness which can be caused by such factors as diabetes, kidney damage or brain damage. For the latter case, it has been known for Reflexology to help where other methods had failed.
DR: brain, head.
AR: spine, heart, kidney, pancreas.

17 Conjunctivitis

This is where the conjunctiva (the membrane lining the eyelids and covering the white portion of the eye) becomes inflamed with redness, itching, swelling and discharge from the eye.
DR: eyes.
AR: upper lymph nodes, kidneys, adrenals, upper spine.

18 Constipation

The term relating to infrequent and difficult evacuation of the bowel. The condition arises from poor muscle tone in the intestines which can result from lack of fibre in the diet, lack of exercise and fatigue and anxiety.
DR: large intestine.
AR: small intestine, adrenals, solar plexus, liver, lower spine.

19 Cough

A cough is a protective reflex aimed at clearing anything which is interfering with the breathing apparatus. A cough may be dry or may include mucus being cleared out from the air passageways.
DR: throat.
AR: bronchi, lungs, upper lymph nodes.

20   Cramp

This is where a muscle or group of muscles goes into spasm remaining contracted and producing great pain. Some people may suffer from frequent bouts of cramp particularly at night. These may be caused by mineral imbalances in the body. For immediate relief of cramp, brisk massage to the affected part is helpful.

DR: area affected.
AR: parathyroids, heart.

21   Cystitis

In this condition the bladder becomes inflamed and infected with resultant pain on passing water and often accompanying lower back and abdominal pain.

DR: bladder.
AR: kidneys, ureter tubes, adrenals, lymph nodes of pelvis, pituitary, prostate.

22   Deafness

Diminished hearing can result from a number of factors including damage to the ear following surgery on the ear, damage to the nerve supply to the ear, deafness due to catarrhal congestion or excessive wax in the ears. Of these, only the first mentioned is unlikely to be helped by treatment.

DR: ears.
AR: side of head, upper spine, neck, sinuses, eustachian tube, solar plexus.

23   Depression

This is an emotional disorder with a lowering of the mental and physical state of the body. The treatment can help improve the general physical state of the body which in turn may help the person mentally. Some form of counselling will also be needed to try to find the cause of the problem.

DR: areas relating to symptoms experienced.
AR: head, brain, pituitary, thyroid, adrenals, reproductive areas, solar plexus.

24 Dermatitis

This is a skin condition, causing inflammation and irritation, which usually begins after contact with an irritating substance either a food or chemical. The condition is easily aggravated by fatigue and stress. Avoidance of the irritating substance is advised.

DR: parts of skin affected.
AR: solar plexus, adrenals, liver, digestive areas, kidneys.

25 Diabetes

This condition involves a metabolic disorder in the body where the ability to utilize carbohydrates is affected. Normally, carbohydrates are broken down into glucose which is the body's principal energy source. The conversion of glucose to energy is controlled by the hormone, insulin, produced by the pancreas. In diabetes, there is insufficient insulin to break down the glucose with a resulting increase in the blood sugar level. The symptoms of diabetes are excessive thirst, frequent passing of urine, increased appetite and loss of weight. With long-term diabetes, the eyes, kidneys and blood vessels may be affected.

EXTREME CARE is necessary when giving Reflexology treatment to a diabetic since the treatment may cause the pancreas to start producing more insulin and if the patient is already taking insulin there will be too much insulin present resulting in the blood sugar level being lowered too much. The diabetic *can* be treated though and if necessary, the pancreas reflex area can be avoided with work on the other areas to help prevent some of the long-term effects of the disorder.

DR: pancreas.
AR: liver, kidneys, eyes, adrenals, pituitary.

26 Diarrhoea

In this condition there is too frequent evacuation of the bowel with the stools being more watery than normal. The condition usually occurs due to dietary factors and sometimes anxiety.

DR: large intestine.
AR: small intestine, liver, solar plexus, adrenals.

27 Diverticulitis

In this condition there is inflammation of the small sacs (called diverticula) found along the small or large intestine walls. The symptoms which can occur include abdominal pains and bloating, a frequent urge to eliminate but followed by constipation. Infection can also be present.
DR: small and large intestine.
AR: adrenals, solar plexus, lymphatic areas.

28 Ear ache

This may occur due to infection in the ear or from being out in severe cold.
DR: ears.
AR: eustachian tubes, upper lymph nodes, side of head, neck, upper spine.

29 Eczema

This skin condition involves inflamed, itching skin with the formation of scales on the skin. It may be related to allergic factors and is usually aggravated by fatigue and stress.
DR: areas to parts of skin affected.
AR: solar plexus, adrenals, kidneys, digestive areas, liver, pituitary.

30 Emphysema

This condition affects the lungs and symptoms of breathlessness and a cough result. These are due to the fact that the elasticity of the air sacs is lost so that having been stretched with breathing in, they are not able to recoil back for breathing out which becomes less effective.
DR: lungs.
AR: adrenals, bronchi, solar plexus, heart.

31 Epilepsy

This condition is characterized by seizures caused by an electrical disturbance in the nerve cells in the brain. Loss of consciousness can occur, as may abnormal behaviour of some muscles.
DR: brain.
AR: solar plexus, spine, digestive areas and endocrine areas.

Extra Care must be taken with treatment of the epileptic since over-stimulation might cause a fit.

32 Eye strain

The eyes can become strained from reading or working in a poor light and when overtired. It has been found that Reflexology treatment can also help improve problems with failing eye sight.
DR: eyes.
AR: solar plexus, adrenals, spine, kidneys.

33 Fibroids

These are quite common, harmless tumours which grow in the uterus and can become quite large. Treatment may cause the fibroid to be dispersed and this will be shed in a manner similar to a period.
DR: uterus.
AR: ovaries, fallopian tubes, pelvic lymphatic areas.

34 Fibrositis

In this condition there is pain and stiffness with resulting limitation of movement in muscles and ligaments. The areas most commonly affected are the lower back, neck and shoulders and the trouble can occur from the cold or damp or from unaccustomed movement.
DR: areas which are affected.
AR: solar plexus, adrenals.

35 Flatulence

Also known as wind, this results from an accumulation of gas in the digestive tract which is either released upwards from the stomach or downwards from the large intestine. In the stomach it is often caused by swallowing air, dietary factors and stress and in the large intestine it is caused by faulty bowel movement either as constipation or diarrhoea.
DR: stomach or large intestine.
AR: digestive areas, solar plexus, diaphragm, liver.

36 Foot problems

Some foot problems may be helped by the general treatment given to the foot though obviously care must be taken if the foot is seriously injured. Poor muscle tone and tension in the feet can be eased and sometimes structural problems with the foot can be corrected.
DR: corresponding area on hand as zone related area.
AR: adrenals, spine, solar plexus.

37 Fractures

The healing of a complete break or fracture of a bone can be helped by treatment.
DR: area affected, direct massage to zone related area, e.g. massage the ankle to help a broken wrist.
AR: associated areas to where fracture has occurred, spine, adrenals, solar plexus, parathyroids.

38 Frozen shoulder

In this condition the shoulder joint becomes stiff and painful and can lead to the arm not being able to be moved, hence the term 'frozen'. The pain can spread across the back and the chest as well as down the arm.
DR: shoulder.
AR: shoulder girdle, arm, neck, upper spine, adrenals, solar plexus.

39 Gall stones

Small stones made up of cholesterol, calcium and bile pigments are formed if the bile becomes overconcentrated by the gall bladder. These stones can be passed without problem by passing out from the gall bladder, down the bile duct and into the duodenum. If, however, the stones are large they may block the bile duct and this can lead to inflammation of the gall bladder and jaundice. With treatment, it may be possible to help small stones to be passed.

DR: gall bladder.

AR: bile duct (linking gall bladder to duodenum), small intestine, liver, solar plexus, adrenals.

40 Glaucoma

This condition involves the eyes and results in the surface of the eyeball becoming hardened due to an increased pressure of the fluid within the eyeball. The symptoms will include pain in the eyes with blurred vision and halos around lights with also a loss of vision at the sides. In serious cases, glaucoma can lead to blindness.

DR: eyes.

AR: head, upper spine, kidneys.

41 Goitre

This is a swelling of the thyroid gland which will be seen and felt in the front of the neck. In some instances, it may affect swallowing and breathing. It can be due to an iodine deficiency, infection of the thyroid gland or over- or under-production of the thyroid hormones.

DR: thyroid.

AR: pituitary, adrenals, reproductive areas, neck.

42 Gout

In gout there is a metabolic disturbance causing an excess of uric acid in the blood and uric acid salts can settle around the joints, especially the fingers and toes. The affected joint becomes extremely painful, shiny, swollen and red. Dietary factors often contribute to this disorder.
DR: area affected, if big toe then thumb joint would be treated as zone related area.
AR: solar plexus, adrenals, kidneys, liver, parathyroids, pituitary.

43 Haemorrhoids

These are varicose veins (also known as piles) formed in the rectum and usually occur as a result of persistent constipation. There may be discomfort in the area and blood passed with the stools.
DR: rectum.
AR: large intestine, small intestine, liver, heart.

44 Hay fever

This is an allergic reaction to pollen and, when the pollen count is high, hay fever sufferers will show the symptoms of catarrh, a streaming nose, sore throat and excessive watering of the eyes, and also sneezing. The treatment can help by reducing the over-sensitivity of the areas affected and thus relieving the symptoms.
DR: sinuses, eyes, throat, nose.
AR: adrenals, head, digestive areas.

45 Headaches

Most people suffer from a headache at some time but more regular occurrence of headaches may be related to problems such as sinus trouble, eye problems, allergies or tension.
DR: head.
AR: eyes, upper spine, neck, sinuses, digestive area, liver, solar plexus.

46 Heart attack

This can be identified by a sudden, severe pain in the chest which may well radiate up to the left shoulder and down the left arm. There is a feeling of great tightness in the chest and breathlessness. The condition occurs due to an insufficient blood supply to the coronary (heart) muscles which occurs due to thickening of the walls of the arteries caused by fatty deposits consisting mainly of cholesterol. Parts of this may flake off and form a blockage in the already narrowed channel of the artery and a clot can form (thrombosis) if the artery wall is rough or damaged. Recovery is possible from a heart attack but if precautionary measures are not taken, then the likelihood of reoccurence is quite great.

EXTRA CARE should be taken when treating the heart reflex area in all persons with a heart problem due to the risk of overstimulation.
DR: heart.
AR: shoulder, arm, solar plexus, adrenals, digestive areas.

47 Hepatitis

In this condition there is inflammation of the liver due to a virus. The symptoms will be fever, a distaste for food, diarrhoea and vomiting. Hepatitis is usually followed by jaundice.
DR: liver.
AR: lymphatic areas, spleen, stomach, small intestine, large intestine, pituitary.

48 Hernia

A hernia is an abnormal protrusion of an abdominal organ through a weakness in the abdominal muscular wall. The most common sites for a hernia are in the groin (inguinal hernia) and where the oesophagus passes through the diaphragm (hiatus hernia). A hernia will cause discomfort in the region affected.
DR: diaphragm, stomach or groin, large intestine.
AR: oesophagus, solar plexus, adrenals.

49 Hypertension

The term 'hyper' means above, the opposite of this being 'hypo' meaning below. Hypertension means too much tension and the term is used to describe high blood pressure. One of the main causes of high blood pressure is tension and other causes may include obesity, too much salt in the diet, excessive drinking of tea, coffee, alcohol and other stimulants and smoking. The symptoms of high blood pressure are sometimes not that obvious but may include headaches, insomnia, nose bleeds, dizziness and noises in the ears, blurred vision, shortness of breath, oedema and nervousness. People with high blood pressure should try to follow a less stressful life.

DR: heart.

AR: solar plexus, adrenals, kidneys, head, eyes, lungs, neck, spine.

50 Hypoglycaemia

In this condition there is a decreased blood sugar level and this can be caused by too much sugar in the diet which will stimulate the pancreas to produce an excess of insulin. This excess of insulin removes too much sugar from the blood leading to an abnormally low blood sugar level. This condition may also be related to pancreas and liver disorders. The symptoms which may be present are fatigue, weakness in the legs, swollen feet, tightness in the chest, migraine, eyeache, hunger, general pains in the body, mental disturbances and insomnia. Mild forms of this disorder can be quite common due to the high intake of sugar in the diet of many people nowadays.

DR: pancreas, liver.

AR: head, brain, eyes, adrenals, solar plexus, areas to joints and limbs.

51   Hypotension

This refers to the condition where there is a low blood pressure. The symptoms experienced may include fatigue, a lack of endurance, a sensitivity to cold and heat, the need for more sleep and a rapid pulse after exertion. The person may often feel more tired in the morning than before they went to bed. Stress can also contribute to this disorder as well as imbalances of the adrenal glands.

DR: heart.
AR: solar plexus, adrenals, kidneys, head, brain.

52   Incontinence

This refers to an inability to control the passing of water and will involve a problem with the bladder. There may be weakness of the bladder muscles. The term will also cover bedwetting in young children which is often also associated with emotional factors.

DR: bladder.
AR: kidneys, ureter tubes, solar plexus, adrenals, spine, prostate, pituitary.

53   Indigestion

This can also be termed dyspepsia and refers to an incomplete digestion of foods in the stomach or intestines. This will result in abdominal pains and a sense of fullness and discomfort and may be accompanied by gas in the stomach or intestines. It can be caused by overeating and eating too quickly or when under stress, and certain foods may be more likely to produce the condition.

DR: stomach, intestines.
AR: solar plexus, diaphragm.

54 Infection

Infections occur when bacteria or viruses invade the body and the body's defence systems are not able to fight them off. The healthy body has a strong defence system but when there is insufficient resistance offered due to the body being in a low state of health then infection can set in at any point in the body. With serious infections standard medical treatment will be required but Reflexology can be helpful in clearing mild infections and also in strengthening the body to fight off infections more readily.

DR: areas to parts affected.

AR: lymphatic areas, spleen, adrenals, liver, kidneys, pituitary.

55 Infertility

This means a failure to conceive, and the problem may be with the man or the woman or due to slight weaknesses in both. In any case, the problem may involve hormonal imbalances or disorders affecting the reproductive glands.

DR: testes, prostate or ovaries, fallopian tubes, uterus.

AR: pituitary, thyroid, lymphatic areas.

56 Insomnia

An inability to sleep which may involve difficulty in getting off to sleep, waking during the night or waking early and then not returning to sleep. All people have different sleep needs and some people can manage with very much less sleep than others. Usually, with age less sleep is required. The problem of insomnia may be due to physical symptoms which produce pain and thus keep the person awake or waken them but often the problem is due to psychological factors, the commonest of which are probably stress and anxiety.

DR: brain.

AR: solar plexus, areas where physical pain present.

57 Jaundice

In jaundice there is yellowness of the skin and the whites of the eyes due to the presence of bile pigments in the blood. This can be caused by a liver problem, a blocked bile duct or infection spreading from the intestines. It may also indicate a blood or kidney disorder.

DR: liver, gall bladder.

AR: small intestine, lymphatic areas, spleen, kidneys, pituitary.

58 Knee pains

Knee pains may be due to sprains, pulled ligaments, damage to the cartilage of the knee, or arthritis. In these cases, there may be both pain and inflammation of one or both joints.

DR: knee.

AR: elbow (massage directly as zone related area), adrenals, parathyroids, solar plexus, spine, hip.

59 Kidney stones

These stones are formed in the kidney and consist mainly of calcium. They can be deposited either in the kidney or in the ureter tube. Great pain will be experienced, starting in the middle back and radiating around the abdomen towards the groin. There may be increased urination and nausea and vomiting. It is also possible that a kidney stone can set up infection in the urinary tract.

DR: kidneys.

AR: ureter tube, bladder, lymphatic areas, parathyroids, lumbar spine, pituitary, adrenals.

60 Lumbago

This is where there is a pain in the lower back in the region of the lumbar spine. The problem may be due to sprains of the muscles or ligaments in the lumbar region or damage to the intervertebral discs in this region.

DR: spine (lumbar region).

AR: solar plexus, adrenals.

61 Mastitis

In this condition there is inflammation of the breast and there will be pain or discomfort felt in one or both breasts. It may occur just prior to a period or after straining the arm or from damage to the breast tissue.
DR: breast.
AR: lymphatic areas, adrenals, arm.

62 Ménière's disease

This condition involves the inner ear and will produce symptoms of deafness, giddiness, noises in the ear, nausea and vomiting.
DR: ears.
AR: head, eustachian tubes, neck, upper spine, stomach, pituitary.

63 Meningitis

In this condition there is inflammation of the meninges which are the membranes surrounding the brain and the spinal cord. The symptoms present will include a bad headache, a stiff neck, a high fever, nausea, vomiting and changes in body temperature. The condition should be treated by a medical practitioner but during the recovery period, Reflexology may be of help.
DR: brain, spine.
AR: head, pituitary, lymphatic areas, spleen.

64 Menopause

This is the cessation of menstruation which occurs in women between about 40 and 50 years. It can pass without any noticeable symptoms but in some women considerable problems can occur including hot flushes, headaches, dizziness, mood changes, digestive disturbances and irregular periods with heavy bleeding. Treatment can sometimes prevent the need for a hysterectomy which may be required if there are problems with the menopause.
DR: ovaries, fallopian tubes, uterus, pituitary.
AR: thyroid, adrenals, head, ears, digestive areas.

65 Menstrual problems

Menstruation is the flow of blood from the uterus which occurs once a month in women from about the age of 12 or 13 until the menopause at the age of 40 to 50. Various problems can be associated with menstruation including heavy periods, scanty periods, an absence of periods, irregular periods, pain at the time of a period and pre-menstrual tension which refers to the normal physiological and psychological changes which occur at the time of menstruation but can become exaggerated and troublesome. The problems are all associated with the hormonal changes which take place at this time.

DR: ovaries, uterus.
AR: pituitary, thyroid, adrenals, fallopian tubes, solar plexus, head.

66 Migraine

A migraine is a severe headache which can be accompanied by visual disturbances, nausea, vomiting and even speech difficulties. It can be caused by a number of different factors including an allergy to certain foods, eyestrain, tension, neck problems, hormonal problems and sinus congestion.

DR: head.
AR: neck, spine, eyes, sinuses, pituitary, thyroid, ovaries, digestive areas, liver, solar plexus.

67   Multiple Sclerosis

This is a condition affecting the protective covering of the nerves in the brain and spinal cord which results in hardening of various parts of the nervous system and the development of scars or lesions on the affected nerves. The cause of the disease is not fully known but may be associated with nutritional imbalances, infection or even stress. The symptoms may include visual and speech disturbances, dizziness, loss of balance, lack of co-ordination, paralysis, bowel and bladder disorders and emotional instability. The disease progresses slowly and remission periods can occur when there is an apparent loss of symptoms.

DR: head, spine.
AR: eyes, ears, intestines, bladder, solar plexus, adrenals, lymphatic areas.

68   Muscle strains

A muscle can be strained by being overused or used in a manner to which it is unaccustomed. This can result in temporary pain and discomfort. Treatment may help to speed up the healing process but resting the muscle is also advised.

DR: area affected, direct massage to zone related area.
AR: solar plexus, adrenals, parathyroids.

69   Neck stiffness

This can be caused by tension, arthritis in the cervical spine, swollen glands, sleeping in a cramped position, turning the head badly or from being in a draught. Problems with the neck can lead to other problems involving, for example, the shoulder, the arm, headaches and ear problems.

DR: neck, cervical spine.
AR: shoulder, arm, head, ears, solar plexus, adrenals.

70 Nephritis

This condition is where there is inflammation of one or both kidneys
resulting from kidney infection. The symptoms may include lower back
pain, a frequent urge to pass water, oedema, fever, chills, nausea,
vomiting and loss of appetite.
DR: kidneys.
AR: ureter tubes, bladder, lymphatic areas, pituitary, lower spine.

71 Neuralgia

This is a general term which means pain in a nerve. The term is often
used to describe trigeminal neuralgia which affects the trigeminal nerve
which supplies the face and this will produce symptoms of severe pain
in the face, the temple, the jaw, the teeth, the ear with possible twitching
of the face muscles on the side affected and watering of the eye. It can
be brought on by the cold.
DR: face.
AR: head, brain, eyes, ears, teeth, solar plexus, upper spine.

72 Ovarian cysts

A cyst is a small sac enclosing fluid or semi-solid matter and one of
the more common sites of formation in the body is the ovary. Treatment
can sometimes cause a cyst to be dispersed and this will appear as a
discharge similar to that of a period. With an ovarian cyst, discomfort
and pain will be felt in the abdomen which may be noticeably swollen.
DR: ovaries.
AR: fallopian tubes, uterus, lymphatic areas.

73 Paralysis

This is where there is a complete or partial loss of nervous function to
a part of the body. This can occur in any part of the body and may involve
local damage to a nerve or damage at the higher nerve centres in the
spinal cord or brain.
DR: area affected.
AR: brain, spine, areas associated with affected part.

74 Parkinson's disease

In this condition there is damage to a part of the brain with resulting effects on the muscular system causing rigidity and cramping in the muscles and involuntary muscle movements, particularly of the hands. The face develops a rather 'mask-like' look and the mouth tends to remain open with an increased production of watery saliva. There can be a tendency for the person to lean forward and to walk with short, shuffling steps. Speech may also be affected and there may be loss of appetite, loss of weight and constipation.
DR: brain, areas affected.
AR: spine, parathyroids, adrenals, digestive areas.

75 Phlebitis

This is an inflammation of the wall of a vein and is usually found in the legs, often as a complication of varicose veins. There will be severe pain in the area affected and reddening and swelling of the vein. There may also be a slight fever.

EXTRA CARE should be taken with the treatment of this condition because of the risk of thrombophlebitis developing which is the formation of a clot in the inflamed vein.
DR: area affected, direct massage to zone related area to part affected.
AR: heart, intestines, pituitary, adrenals.

76 Pleurisy

This is an inflammation of the pleura which are the two thin layers surrounding the lungs. It can produce pain in the side and in the shoulder which is aggravated by coughing. It can occur following a cold or chill or when the lung is inflamed and can sometimes result from general illness in the body such as kidney disease, blood poisoning or ear trouble.
DR: lungs.
AR: lymphatic areas, shoulder, kidneys, ears, adrenals.

77 Pregnancy

This is not of course a disorder but problems can arise during pregnancy which can sometimes be helped by Reflexology. For instance, such problems as morning sickness, constipation, heartburn and kidney infection.

EXTRA CARE must be taken when treating a pregnant woman particularly in the early stages of a first pregnancy or where there have been previous miscarriages.

DR: areas affected, e.g. stomach, intestines, kidneys.
AR: pituitary, thyroids, adrenals, ovaries, uterus.

78 Pre-menstrual tension

This refers to an accentuation of the normal physiological and psychological changes which occur just before a period in women, and includes such symptoms as fatigue, headaches, backache, abdominal pains, constipation, soreness of the breasts, enlarged varicose veins, spots on the face, lack of concentration, irritability and depression. Symptoms can last for several days and are due to the hormonal changes taking place at this time.

DR: areas affected.
AR: ovaries, fallopian tubes, uterus, pituitary, thyroid, adrenals, solar plexus.

79 Prostate gland enlargement

It is not uncommon particularly as men get older, for the prostate gland to enlarge, and this then presses on the bladder, causing a more frequent need to pass water. This becomes particularly noticeable at night and leads to a disturbed sleep. There may also be difficulty in passing water.

DR: prostate.
AR: bladder, ureter tubes, kidneys, lymphatic areas.

80   Psoriasis

This is a skin condition characterized by irregularly-shaped, slightly
raised red patches covered by silvery scales. There need not be much
irritation. The sites most commonly affected are the elbows, knees and
scalp though it can occur on any part of the body. The nails may also
become pitted and ridged. The condition is often made worse by stress.
DR: areas to parts of skin affected.
AR: adrenals, kidneys, liver, digestive areas, solar plexus, pituitary.

81   Raynaud's disease

In this condition the circulatory system is at fault and involves a tightening
of the arteries to the hands and, less often, the feet when they are cooled
resulting in the fingers becoming white and then turning red and swollen.
On getting warm, the fingers will go bright red and patchy with a burning
and tingling sensation.
DR: toes (as zone related area).
AR: heart, digestive areas, liver, endocrine areas, kidneys.

82   Rheumatism

This is a general term used to describe a range of conditions affecting
connective tissue and therefore presenting the symptoms of pain, stiffness
or swelling of muscles and joints. It will cover conditions such as
rheumatic fever, rheumatoid arthritis, anklyosing spondylitis, non-
articular rheumatism, osteoarthritis and gout. The term is usually used
however to describe muscle aches and pains which can occur after getting
wet or cold or using muscles in an unaccustomed manner and most often
affects the lower back and the neck and across the shoulders.
DR: areas affected.
AR: joints associated with areas affected, parathyroids, adrenals.

83 Rhinitis

In this condition there is inflammation of the nasal membranes leading to nasal congestion and an increased secretion of mucus. It can be caused by an allergy such as to pollen (hay fever) or substances such as house dust, feathers, wool, mould or certain foods. If the condition is due to an allergy it may be possible with treatment to reduce the sensitivity of the nasal membranes and thus reduce the reaction caused.

DR: sinuses, nose.

AR: head, spine, eyes, eustachian tube, adrenals, digestive areas.

84 Sciatica

In this condition there is inflammation of the sciatic nerve which is the largest nerve in the body and arises from the lower lumbar and sacral regions of the spine and then passes down across the buttock, down the back of the leg and divides into two main branches just behind and above the knee. With sciatica, pain can be felt along all or part of the pathway of the nerve and there may also be pins and needles or a feeling of numbness along all or part of the pathway of the nerve. The trouble can be caused by several different factors including lower back problems, tilting of the pelvis, hip problems, swelling of the abdomen as in obesity or pregnancy.

DR: sciatic loop and area up back of leg.

AR: lower spine, sacro-iliac joint, muscles of pelvis, hip, knee.

85 Shingles

This condition is caused by a virus which attacks sensory nerves
producing severe pain and the appearance of blisters along the part of
the nerve affected. It is also known as herpes zoster, and the virus
involved is possibly the same as that which causes chicken pox hence
adults can sometimes catch shingles from a child with chicken pox and
vice versa. The areas most commonly affected are the chest, trunk and
face including the eye and usually only one part and one side is affected.
The blisters disappear after about one week but the pain can persist at
intervals for a considerable time. Treatment can be used to help clear
the condition when it is present or to help remove the persistent pain
occurring some time after the blisters have disappeared.

DR: area affected.

AR: lymphatic areas, spleen, solar plexus.

86 Sinusitis

In this condition there is inflammation of the sinuses with resulting pain
and throbbing in the face, a blocked nose, nasal discharge, headaches,
possibly fever and the voice can become husky or nasal. It can occur
following a cold or influenza and can also be caused by allergies or
deformity of the nasal septum.

DR: sinuses, nose.

AR: head, face, eyes, upper lymph nodes, adrenals, neck, upper spine.

87 Spondylitis

This condition refers to inflammation of one or more of the vertebrae
of the spine. In ankylosing spondylitis, the vertebra become stiff and
fixed in position. This will result in pain in the region of the spine affected
and limitation of the normal movements.

DR: spine.

AR: neck, shoulder, arm (if upper spine affected), sacro-iliac joint, pelvic
muscles, hips, sciatic (if lower back affected), adrenals, solar plexus.

88   Stroke

This is the general term used for a cerebral haemorrhage when a blood clot develops on one side of the brain in the cerebrum causing a partial or total paralysis of the opposite side of the body. As well as the upper and lower limbs, speech can also be affected and the person may suffer from confusion. Recovery from a stroke can occur and can be helped by treatment even some years after the stroke occurred.

DR: head, brain, areas affected (upper limb, lower limb, face).
AR: spine, heart, adrenals.

89   Tear duct blockage

The tears are the natural cleansing agents of the eyes and if the tear ducts become blocked, the eyes will be more irritated by dust and dirt and infection is more likely to occur. If the tear ducts are blocked the eyes will also feel sore and by rubbing the eyes, the person will make the irritation worse.

DR: eyes.
DR: sinuses, head, spine, kidney.

90   Tennis elbow

In this condition there is a pain felt in the outer side of the elbow and sometimes also in the forearm after certain movements of the arm. It occurs not only from playing tennis but also from any action involving the rotation of the forearm. The condition is often aided by rest.

DR: elbow, knee (as zone related area).
AR: arm, shoulder, neck.

91 Tenosynovitis

This condition involves inflammation of the thin synovial lining of a
tendon sheath. A tendon is an inelastic cord which attaches a muscle
to a bone. The term is often used in reference to inflammation of a tendon
in the wrist with resulting swelling and stiffness of the fingers which
tend to remain in a curled position. There may also be numbness and
tingling in the thumb and finger with pain in the palm or forearm. This
condition can be caused by overusing the wrist joint in an unaccustomed
manner, though in some cases may be due to infection.
DR: ankle and toes (as zone related areas).
AR: arm, shoulder, neck, spine, adrenals.

92 Tension

A very large percentage of the different disorders which people develop
can be attributed to tension or stress. The body is able to cope with a
certain amount of stress but with the increased pressures which are placed
on people by contemporary lifestyle, the demands of the body cannot
always be met and ill-health results. Tension can affect any part or parts
of the body resulting in such symptoms as headaches, digestive problems,
backache, neck pains, menstrual and other hormonal imbalances and
allergy conditions. The ability to relax is essential for the well-being
of the whole body and this will reduce any symptoms of tension.
DR: areas affected.
AR: solar plexus, adrenals, pituitary.

93 Thrombosis

This is the formation of a blood clot in the circulatory system. It can
occur in the legs as a complication of phlebitis (inflammation of the veins
– see above), in the brain as in a stroke, in the lungs as in a pulmonary
embolism or in the heart as in a coronary thrombosis. The effect is that
the clot can block the blood flow to the area where it is formed or can
lodge in a blood vessel elsewhere in the body and prevent the blood flow

to that area. This can result in serious or fatal effects. Blood clots are more likely to occur in the walls of blood vessels which have become furred up due to the deposits of fatty materials on the vessel walls.

EXTREME CARE should be taken in the treatment of any person who is at risk from thrombosis. Reflexology treatment can be used to improve circulation and if a person has suffered from a thrombosis, then treatment can be used to help improve recovery.

DR: area affected.
AR: heart, digestive system.

94 Thyroid imbalance

The condition of hyper- or hypo-thyroidism means respectively overactivity or underactivity of the thyroid gland. In the overactive state, the condition of thyrotoxicosis occurs, with the symptoms of a high pulse rate, palpitations, warm skin, excessive perspiration, a large appetite but without weight gain, nervousness, tremor and protruding eyes. It can be associated with a goitre (thyroid swelling) since the extra tissue produces extra hormone. In the underactive state, the condition of myxoedema occurs, with weight gain, tiredness, loss of hair, puffiness of the face and eyelids and a feeling of cold at all times.

Treatment is the same with Reflexology whether the gland is over or underactive.

DR: thyroid.
AR: pituitary, adrenals, reproductive areas, eyes.

95 Tinnitus

In this condition there is a ringing, buzzing or thumping noise experienced in one or both ears. The cause of the condition may involve inflammation of the delicate ear mechanism, catarrhal congestion or degeneration of the nerve endings in the ear.

DR: ears.
AR: eustachian tubes, sides of head, neck, upper spine, solar plexus.

96 Tonsillitis

In this condition there is inflammation of the tonsils in the throat. The throat becomes sore, red and swollen and there may be a difficulty in swallowing. The infection may also be accompanied by headaches, earaches and fever.

DR: throat, upper lymph nodes.
AR: lymphatic areas, spleen, head, ears, eustachian tube, pituitary.

97 Toothache

Pain in the teeth can sometimes be relieved by treatment but if persistent, a dentist should always be consulted. The reflex areas will relate not only to the teeth but also to the gums around the teeth. It has been known for Reflexology to be used in place of an anaesthetic for dental treatment by applying pressure to the appropriate zones in the hands.

DR: teeth (affected zone).
AR: face, solar plexus.

98 Ulcers

An ulcer is an open sore on the skin or mucous membrane. If an ulcer is formed in the stomach it is called a peptic ulcer and if formed in the first part of the small intestine it is called a duodenal ulcer. Both of these conditions can cause pain in the upper abdominal regions with a feeling of fullness which is often relieved by food. These conditions can be associated with stress and an unsuitable diet. A varicose ulcer is a skin ulcer commonly found on the inner side of the lower part of the leg near the ankle associated with varicose veins. This type of ulcer can be very painful and can take a considerable length of time to heal.

DR: area affected (stomach, duodenum, skin).
AR: digestive areas, massage direct to zone related area for skin ulcer, heart.

99   Varicose veins

These are veins that become enlarged, twisted and swollen and they are most commonly found in the legs and, in the first instance, usually the lower leg. The condition can be caused by a disorder of the valves in the veins or from a lower abdominal swelling such as in pregnancy or obesity which affects the back flow of blood from the veins of the legs. It is unlikely that treatment will cause the disappearance of varicose veins but it can often help the associated discomfort and also help to prevent a worsening of the condition.

DR: areas affected, direct massage to zone related area.
AR: heart, digestive areas, abdominal areas (if distended).

100   Vertigo

In this condition there is dizziness and giddiness and a sensation of spinning or a feeling that the ground is rising and falling. Vertigo may also be accompanied by nausea, vomiting, headaches and perspiration. It is caused by an imbalance in the functioning of the inner ear which may be due to infection, injury or other imbalances in the body.

DR: ears.
AR: head, eustachian tubes, sinuses, neck, upper spine, solar plexus.

8 Examples of Treatment

As evidence of the effectiveness of Reflexology treatment, the following examples are of courses of treatment which have been given and the results which have been achieved. Although headed under a specific disorder, you will see that in most instances the person being treated had several things affecting them, though initially they sought treatment for one main problem. In many instances, the other problems were also corrected or helped.

Allergies

A woman had suffered with digestive problems including vomiting and severe abdominal pains for 24 years. After many tests when nothing could be found to be wrong, it was discovered that this lady suffered from numerous food allergies. By adjusting her diet and being very careful about what she ate, the symptoms had been much improved. This lady came for treatment since, although her symptoms had improved, they were still present and she felt that Reflexology might help. At the first treatment session her feet were quite sensitive, particularly in the regions of the big toes, the right ear and Eustachian tube (the woman reported that she was deaf in her right ear), the solar plexus, the liver, the small intestine, the large intestine (which was the most tender reflex area), the kidney and adrenal areas. As her feet were worked on, the woman described a feeling of a 'flow of energy' up from her feet throughout her body. Similar areas were found to be tender for the next two treatments which followed at weekly intervals but she noticed no improvement of the symptoms. The woman then thought she would stop the treatment but a week later rang to say that she was feeling so much better that she felt she should have some further treatments. Her symptoms involving the digestive system had disappeared as had the majority of her food allergies and although still following a sensible diet she had been able to eat foods which she had not been able to tolerate for years including a glass of wine. In addition, she had found that the pain which she had had in her lower back for some time had also disappeared and she was delighted with her improvement.

Asthma

A teenage girl had for five years suffered from asthma and, to a lesser extent, eczema. The asthma mainly affected her if she ran about or when the weather was wet. She caught a lot of colds which were always followed by a cough which persisted. At the first treatment session, the reflex areas in the feet were not very sensitive though a slight tenderness was felt in the regions of the big toes, the reflexes of the sinuses, the lungs, the solar plexus, the kidneys and adrenals. In the week following the first treatment, the patient reported that she had sneezed a lot and often needed to blow her nose, both of which were probably a result of the treatment. Treatment continued at weekly intervals and at the fourth session, the young girl reported that she was feeling much better and had used her inhaler on very few occasions. By the seventh session, the improvement was even more noticeable and the girl had been able to take much more exercise without ill effects. There was still slight tendernesses felt in the feet when the reflex areas were massaged though at no time during the course of treatment did the feet appear very tender.

Backache

A middle-aged woman had experienced a Reflexology treatment whilst staying with her sister and since it had helped to ease the backache which she was experiencing she decided to follow a course of treatment. The back problem had been present for ten years with the pain in the lower back and right hip. She had consulted an osteopath which had helped her slightly and she did regular exercises for her back but the pain was present for most of the time and particularly bad if she did much exercise such as walking or gardening or if she carried anything quite heavy. At the first treatment session, many tender areas were found including those

of the big toes, the reflexes to the sinuses, eyes (the lady suffered from
headaches, a sinus problem and sore eyes), the neck, the solar plexus,
the small intestines, the ileo-caecal valve (this was particularly tender
and the woman reported having a problem with constipation), the large
intestine and rectum, the lower spine, the right hip, the right sacro-iliac
joint and the pelvic muscles on the right side. With subsequent treatments,
the reflex areas became less tender and the woman noticed that she was
feeling much less tense. After four treatments, the back problem was
greatly improved and the woman then decided to have treatment at
monthly intervals. After three months, she said that she was feeling much
better with no back pain and she had been walking to work each morning,
which took about half an hour, with no bad effects. Her sinuses were
clearer, her eyes no longer sore and she was now only occasionally
troubled by constipation or headaches.

Chilblains

A woman in her thirties came for treatment during the winter since her
health had not picked up following a bad bout of 'flu. She was normally
in quite good health with no specific problems though she did have a
poor circulation with very cold feet and in the winter always suffered
from chilblains on her toes. At the first treatment session, her feet were
found to be extremely cold. The reflex areas were quite tender especially
those to the neck, sinuses, solar plexus, heart, liver, large intestine,
kidneys and adrenals. This woman had three weekly treatment sessions
by which time she reported that she was feeling back to her normal
energetic self with a greatly improved circulation to her feet – she could
not remember ever having warm feet and no chilblains, especially in
the winter, but this was now the case.

Constipation

A middle-aged man decided to try Reflexology treatment to see if it could
help his long-standing problem of constipation. He also had a problem
with catarrh and his nose always felt blocked even though he seemed to
have to blow it a lot. He had a course of six treatments at regular, weekly,
intervals during which time the reflex areas in the feet appeared to be

quite sensitive particularly those in the big toes, to the sinuses, the neck, the lower back, the liver, the small intestine and the large intestine including the ileo-caecal valve. After the first treatment session, the catarrh began to clear and the man experienced a good deal of discharge from the nose, similar to a heavy cold. As treatment progressed, his bowel movements became more regular and after six weeks, the man reported that his head and nose were no longer blocked and that the problem of constipation was greatly improved. He was having a regular daily bowel movement, whereas previously the bowels had only been evacuated every three or four days. This man was also encouraged to maintain the high-fibre diet which assisted his improvement.

Cystitis

A 50-year-old woman had had recurring cystitis for many years and for the past two years had had loss of control of the emptying of the bladder. She also suffered from headaches which she thought were associated with the menopause and stress due to family problems. The reflex areas in her feet at the first treatment session were quite sensitive and in particular those to the pituitary, head, neck, lower spine, small intestine, bladder, uterer tubes, kidneys, adrenals, ovaries, lymphatics and solar plexus. With subsequent treatments, the reflex areas became less sensitive though the woman was not able to report any improvement. However, at the fifth treatment she said that the cystitis had cleared and that her control over the emptying of the bladder was also much better. She said that she was feeling much better in herself and although her family problems had become worse, she was coping with the additional stress much better than she could have imagined.

Depression

A woman came for treatment to help with depression which had arisen following the death of her mother. She did not really have any physical symptoms apart from the occasional headache and not sleeping well, but she generally felt low in vitality. At the first treatment session, her feet appeared to be sensitive in most of the areas but particularly the big toes, neck and solar plexus. As weekly treatments progressed, the feet were still very sensitive and she reported feeling a little better. By the fifth treatment the woman was delighted with her improvement: she was coping better, was sleeping better and had even been out shopping by herself which she had not managed to do for months. There then followed a slight return of the depression following a car accident but with a few more treatments she was back to what she considered to be her normal self.

Frozen shoulder

A woman had suffered from a frozen shoulder which was accompanied by pins and needles down the right arm and into the hand. The problem had been present for about a year and had not responded to hospital treatment though there had been a slight improvement in her shoulder condition. The reflex areas in her feet were not very sensitive but extra massage was given to those areas relating to the neck, right shoulder and shoulder girdle and right arm. After three treatments the woman said that there was much less pain in the shoulder but still the pins and needles in the arm. By the sixth treatment, both her shoulder and her arm were feeling much better and this woman continued with treatment for nine sessions by which time she had no more pain in the shoulder or arm and also said that she was sleeping better.

Hay fever

A young girl was brought for Reflexology treatment during the spring to try and reduce the problem which she experienced with hay fever in the summer. She also seemed to be allergic to house dust, feathers, and cats, all of which produced, like the hay fever, sneezing, a runny nose and a blocked nose. During the first treatment session, the girl sneezed a lot and was having to blow her nose most of the time. The reflex areas in her feet were not very sensitive but there was a slight tenderness felt in the areas to the head, sinuses, neck, intestines, kidneys and adrenals. The girl said how much she had enjoyed the treatment and had previously been worried that it might be very painful. After the first treatment, she was very much worse for a few days but then the symptoms eased. By the second treatment she was looking much better and at the third session reported that she had been very well since the last treatment, with a lessening of her symptoms. She then discontinued with treatment but her mother reported that the following summer, when the pollen count had been quite high, the girl had had very few problems and was hardly affected at all.

Insomnia

A woman came for treatment for arthritis in the neck, shoulders and back and also mentioned that she had bad insomnia. She only managed to sleep for a few hours at night and never managed to sleep at all during the day. This woman had rather tough feet but they were fairly sensitive in the areas relating to the pituitary, neck, upper and lower spine, shoulder and shoulder girdle, parathyroids, solar plexus, stomach, bladder (she occasionally suffered from cystitis), hip and pelvic regions. After the treatment she said that her feet were 'tingling' and she felt very 'light' in the top of the body. At the second treatment session, she said that she had felt very tired after the previous treatment and had had an excellent sleep that night and also most other nights in the week. The pain in her shoulder had also improved. After a course of four, weekly, treatments, the woman was sleeping for about six hours each night and was feeling much better for this. Her shoulder pain was also improved and she decided to continue with regular monthly treatments to ensure that the improvement remained.

Knee pain

A sportsman was suffering from knee pain so decided to try Reflexology treatment. This man was otherwise quite healthy, apart from occasional lower back problems. The reflex areas of his feet were not found to be particularly sensitive except the areas to the knees and lower spine. After the first treatment session, his knees were found to be free of pain but a short course of treatment was followed to prevent the condition returning. This person still suffers from knee problems at intervals, usually as a result of straining the knee during exercise but one or two treatment sessions seems to clear the condition.

Migraine

A middle-aged woman had suffered from migraines since about the age of thirty. These initially occured just before her monthly period but had become more frequent, occurring nearly every two to three weeks and lasting for two or three days. She also suffered from other symptoms related to hormonal imbalance, before her period and had a sinus problem. Her feet at the first treatment session were found to be rather stiff and tense with many tender areas including those of the head, pituitary, neck, shoulders, sinuses, eyes, thyroid, solar plexus, kidneys, adrenals, ovaries and uterus. At the second treatment session a week later, the woman reported that she had not had a bad head that week. Treatment continued for several weeks, during which time the reflex areas in the feet became less sensitive and the woman still did not suffer from a migraine. The interval between treatments was extended to two, three and then four weeks and on the whole the lady remained free of migraines except on a couple of occasions when she was under a lot of stress but even then she only had a slight headache which passed off quickly, rather than a migraine which might have lasted a couple of days.

Neck stiffness

A man had been suffering with pain in the neck and shoulders, more on the left side than the right, for several months and movement of his neck was becoming more difficult. He also had occasional pain in the left hip and lower back on the left side. His feet were not particularly sensitive at the first treatment session but slight discomfort was felt in the areas of the neck, lower spine, shoulders, solar plexus, intestines, sacro-iliac joints and hips. At the second treatment session, the man said that following the first treatment he had had considerable pain in the lower back and hip for two days but this had then passed and he was now free from pain. The feet appeared to be more sensitive at this session and at the third session, the man said that he had been free of pain in the back, hips and neck and that he could now turn his head round more comfortably which was especially noticeable when reversing his car. After four treatments, improvement was maintained and the neck and shoulders were free from pain, and more mobile.

Pre-menstrual tension

A woman in her thirties had been advised by a friend to try Reflexology to help her problem with pre-menstrual tension. For a week before her period was due, the woman would be depressed and irritable and would have severe abdominal pains and painful breasts. Some months her condition was bad enough for her to have to take time off work which worried her. At the first treatment session, the reflex areas to the pituitary, head, neck, sinuses, eustachian tubes, shoulders, kidneys, adrenals, ovaries, uterus and lymphatic system were all quite tender. This woman also added that she was prone to ear infections if she was run down. After treatment she felt very tired and went home and had to go to bed very early. A similar reaction occurred in response to subsequent treatments. After weekly sessions for a period of just over two months, she reported having less problems before her periods and was also feeling much better in herself. Regular treatments at six weekly intervals followed in order to keep the woman in good health now that the main problems had been cleared. She also noted that she had rarely had an ear infection since starting treatment.

Sciatica

A man came for treatment for sciatica. Over the years he had had recurring problems with lower back pain and sciatica and on this occasion had been in severe pain for three days and was unable to stand up straight and had great difficulty sitting down or getting up from a chair. The most comfortable position was to be lying flat. Otherwise, the man was quite healthy apart from a slight sinus problem. His feet were not very sensitive but particular attention was paid to the reflex areas of the lower spine, sacro-iliac joint and surrounding muscles, the sciatic loop and the sciatic area up the back of the leg. By the end of the first treatment, the man was in less pain and able to straighten up. In this case treatment was given twice a week and improvement continued. By the fourth treatment all pain had gone so treatment was ceased. A couple of months later, he returned for treatment since he had again developed back pain and sciatica following a weekend of gardening. Twice weekly treatment was given for a further two weeks and the condition was then righted.

Sinusitis

A lady came for treatment to help a persistent problem with sinusitis. This caused her to have headaches and aching eyes, her eyes becoming bloodshot. In some instances the headaches were severe enough to be termed migraines. This woman's feet were fairly insensitive at the first session but a slight tenderness was felt in the areas of the head, sinuses, eyes, neck, shoulders, solar plexus, liver and lymphatics. The woman felt very relaxed after treatment. By the fourth treatment she was able to say that her sinuses were much clearer and she had not had any headaches or eye problems. Her neck also felt less tense. A course of seven treatments was given by which time the woman was, in her own words, feeling marvellous.

Tear duct blocked

For two years, a woman had had blocked tear ducts following a bad attack of conjunctivitis. She was having to use drops for her eyes which were also very itchy. At the time the problem started she had been rather run down but was generally in good health. The reflex areas in the feet were quite sensitive at the first session, with tenderness felt in the areas of the head, upper spine, neck, sinuses, eyes, parathyroids, kidneys and adrenals. By the second session one week later, she was delighted with her improvement. She had started to form tears again and had not used her eye drops at all. Her eyes also looked much brighter. Treatment continued at weekly intervals during which there was one slight reoccurrence of the problem but it then cleared again.

Thyroid imbalance

A woman in her forties had been told by her doctor that her thyroid gland was slightly overactive. No treatment was recommended but the woman was worried by her symptoms of a rapid pulse, feeling faint and exhausted. She also seemed to perspire more than usual and had food cravings from time to time but no weight gain. At the first session, the reflex areas of the feet were found to be quite sensitive and in particular those areas to the pituitary, head (she experienced some headaches), neck, eyes, thyroid, solar plexus, bladder, kidneys, adrenals, ovaries, uterus, lymphatic system. At the second treatment session, she reported having felt less panicky than before and she felt her heart rate had slowed down. Again the feet were quite sensitive. By the fourth treatment session, the woman was feeling much better and had become more relaxed. Her feet were also less sensitive. One further treatment was given and the woman felt that her improvement was stable even through a few occasions when she had been under extra stress and would normally have not been able to cope.

Tonsillitis

A woman was suffering from recurring bouts of tonsillitis and had a sore throat for most of the time. She also suffered from a catarrh and sinus problem and some digestive problems. At the first treatment session, there was a slight tenderness of the reflex areas of the head, pituitary, neck, throat, sinuses, eustachian tubes, ears, large intestines, solar plexus, kidneys and adrenals. Another treatment was given one week later at which the woman said she was feeling better with more energy and no longer a sore throat. Her feet were more sensitive at this treatment and especially the areas of the neck, ears and upper lymph nodes and throat. At the third session, improvement was still reported and her feet were less sensitive. The woman then discontinued with treatment though it might well have been wise for her to have had a few more treatments to ensure that there was no more tonsillitis and no further sore throats.

Tinnitus

A man in his seventies had developed tinnitus about a year before trying Reflexology treatment. Initially, he had been troubled by a slight deafness in both ears with some pain but then a buzzing noise developed in his right ear. This man was otherwise in quite good health apart from slight tension in the neck and shoulders and he had required an operation on both hips for arthritis. At the first treatment session, the feet were very sensitive and rather tense. A slight discomfort was felt in the areas relating to the head, neck, ears, eustachian tubes, eyes, solar plexus, kidneys and adrenals. Treatment was advised at weekly intervals and at the second treatment session, the man reported that his ears had been much better for four days after treatment but that the noises had then returned. At the third treatment session, the man reported that the noises had been greatly improved and that the ears had been of little trouble to him during the week. Improvement continued with subsequent treatments and as well as the noises in the ear disappearing for most of the time, his hearing improved. This man continued with regular treatment to maintain the improvement and to keep himself in good health.

Vertigo

A woman had recently developed vertigo so decided to try Reflexology treatment to clear the condition before visiting her doctor. This woman also had a problem with her right ear, and arthritis affecting her hands and elbows. The first treatment session showed tender reflex areas to the pituitary, neck, head, ears, eustachian tubes, thyroid (she also had a thyroid problem), parathyroids, solar plexus, shoulders and arms including the elbows. At the second treatment a week later, the woman said that she had felt very tired after the last treatment but then felt a bit better. The vertigo had cleared. Her feet did not show very tender reflex areas. This woman continued with regular treatment to help the thyroid condition and the vertigo did not return.

These examples are of just some of the conditions which can be helped by a course of Reflexology treatment. In most of these cases the people were cleared of the problem about which they sought treatment. The treatment works in such a way that once the problem is corrected this correction should be maintained unless factors such as injury, diet or undue stress intervene. In some of the cases mentioned, the patient continued with regular treatment to maintain an improved state of health and this is extremely sensible as all who follow this pattern would agree on the value of the benefits which they then derive.

9 Other Treatments Involving the Feet and the Hands

When considering treatment involving the feet, most people naturally think of chiropody and it is not unknown for a person to visit a Reflexology practitioner thinking that they will be able to correct a foot malady. Although this is sometimes possible, the chiropodist is the person qualified to deal with problems involving the feet, such as corns, callouses and some structural problems. It is possible, nowadays to find chiropodists who use homeopathic preparations in their treatments which is preferable for those keen to follow a natural approach to treatment. In some instances, where there are serious structural problems, foot problems will need to be treated by an orthopaedic consultant. The Reflexology practitioner works instead on the feet to treat the whole body and to help the imbalances present in the body.

There are some other alternative therapies which may include working on the feet either for the whole treatment or as a part of the treatment. These therapies will include acupuncture, acupressure, shiatsu, aromatherapy, the metamorphic technique, polarity therapy, massage and the Vacuflex system.

Acupuncture/Acupressure/Shiatsu

The ancient Chinese therapy of acupuncture is based on the theory that within the body there exist meridian lines, along which the vital energy (yin and yang) circulates throughout the body. There are 26 main meridians each associated with a different part or function of the body.

Along the meridian lines are areas called acupressure points or acupoints, and by inserting fine needles to puncture the skin at these points, it is possible to balance the flow of energy of 'chi' along the meridian line. Traditionally, there are about 800 acupoints. As with Reflexology, the acupoints required to balance the system may be quite distant from the part of the body out of balance.

The 12 yang meridians start at the top of the head, face and fingertips and descend to the centre of the body; the 12 yin meridians start from the toes and centre of the body and ascend to the head and the fingertips. There are, therefore, acupoints in the hands and the feet but these points and their meridian lines do not correspond to the reflex points and the longitudinal zones used in Reflexology. When giving acupuncture, some of the points in the hands or feet may be used as part of the treatment.

Acupressure and shiatsu are very similar. Acupressure is often called acupuncture without needles since the same meridian lines and acupoints are worked on but instead of applying needles to the points, a firm pressure and sometimes a circular massage movement is used on the points. Shiatsu is of Japanese origin and the word in Japanese means finger pressure. In this method, as in acupressure, the fingers are pressed onto certain pressure points called *tsubos* which are located along the meridian lines. With both these methods, the feet and hands will be worked on in addition to other parts of the body. It may well be that in certain instances when Reflexology massage is given to the hands or feet, the tenderness felt may be due to working on an acupoint or tsubo rather than a reflex point and some of the points present in the hands and feet are the following (see also figures 66 and 67):

a) a point in the depression between the fourth and fifth metatarsals on the top of the foot (gall bladder meridian) for menstrual irregularities, ringing in the ears and foot pain.
b) a point between the second and third toes just below the web between the toes on the top of the foot (stomach meridian) for toothaches, stomach-ache.
c) a point one and a half inches up from the web between the big toe and the second toe on the top of the foot (liver meridian) for headaches, dizziness.

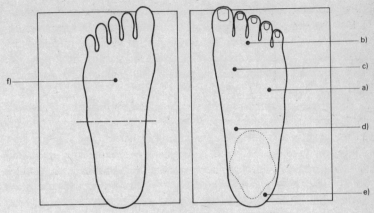

Figure 66   Acupressure points in the feet

d) a point half-way between the front edge of the ankle bone and the extensor muscles on the top of the foot (liver meridian) for arthritis in the ankle.

e) a point between the outer ankle bone and the Achilles tendon (bladder meridian) for sciatica, dizziness, epilepsy.

f) a point on the sole of the foot one third of the way down from the tip of the third toe to the heel (kidney meridian) for epilepsy, dizziness, menstrual irregularities.

g) a point on the outer side of the thumb, one-tenth of an inch to the side from the base of the nail (lung meridian) for sore throats, coughs, pharyngitis, hand spasms, tired arms.

h) a point on the outer side of the top of the wrist below the wrist fold (lung meridian) for breathing problems, cough, pharyngitis.

i) a point on the palm of the hand between the second and third fingers and one inch down from the metacarpophalangeal joint (heart constrictor meridian) for exhaustion.

j) a point between the first and second metacarpals on the back of the hand just below the web between the fingers (large intestine meridian) for diarrhoea, facial tension, rashes and toothache.

k) a point on the second finger on the thumb side, one-tenth of an inch to the side of the base of the nail (large intestine meridian) for diarrhoea and fever.

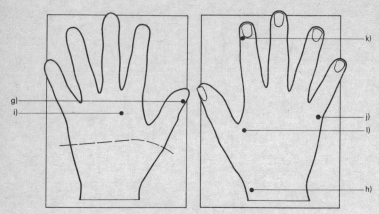

Figure 67   Acupressure points in the hands

l) a point on the back of the hand below the fifth finger at the end of
   the crease which appears when making a fist (small intestine meridian)
   for numbness and paralysis of the fingers, and headaches.

Some of the points of acupressure and shiatsu are sometimes used as
'first-aid' measures and although the idea of balancing up the energy
flow throughout the whole body should be achieved, certainly these points
can in some cases bring relief of minor symptoms.

The presence of meridians in the soles of the feet and how massage
of these meridians could affect the parts of the body to which they related
was described by a Japanese massage teacher, Shizuto Masunaga. These
meridians are shown in figure 68 and the arrows indicate the direction
of the flow of energy in the meridian. By massaging in the direction
of flow of energy, stimulation of the organ occurs; by massaging in the
opposite direction, a calming effect occurs. In order to determine the
duration and effectiveness of this massage, pressure could be applied
to the corresponding reflex points in the feet before and after the massage
to the meridians.

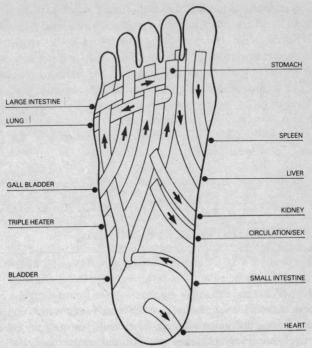

STOMACH

LARGE INTESTINE

LUNG

SPLEEN

LIVER

GALL BLADDER

KIDNEY

TRIPLE HEATER

CIRCULATION/SEX

BLADDER

SMALL INTESTINE

HEART

Figure 68   Meridians in the foot

Aromatherapy

Aromatherapy involves the use of essential oils which are derived from plants. Different oils have different properties and these can be used to treat both physical and emotional conditions. The main use of these essential oils is as massage oils as they dissolve in vegetable oil and are readily absorbed by the skin. The oils are too strong to be used neat.

The therapist selects the appropriate oil for the person to be treated, and massages it into the body with special emphasis on massage to acupressure points helpful to the condition, and to reflex points in the feet. However, the aromatherapy massage is to the whole body and not concentrated on the feet as in Reflexology. Nevertheless, the reflex points can be of great use in this method and the essential oils absorbed through the appropriate reflex points will often enhance the improvement of conditions. Essential oils can also be taken orally and are widely used in cosmetics where their easy absorption and particular actions on the skin can be of great benefit.

The Metamorphic Technique

The metamorphic technique was developed from Reflexology by Robert St John who likened the reflex area to the spine found along the medial border of the foot to the gestation period, the nine months from conception to birth. During the prenatal period, the physical, mental, emotional and spiritual characteristics become established and energy blocks during this time can influence the development of the person. The metamorphic practitioner by working on these reflex areas can act as a catalyst to help improve the energy flow and thus help the energy blocks created during this period.

In relation to the bones of the foot, the areas considered by the practitioner are preconception (from the tip of the toe to the first toe joint), the conception reflex (at the first big toe joint), the post-conception period, the first 18 to 22 weeks (from the first big toe joint to a point midway along the arch of the foot), the quickening reflex (between the medial cuneiform bone and the navicular), the period of pre-birth, from the 18th to 22nd week up to the moment of birth (from the point between the medial cuneiform bone and navicular bone to the top of the calcaneum or heel bone) and the birth reflex (at the top of the heel bone where it meets the Achilles tendon).

With the metamorphic technique, the practitioner will massage, with the tips of the fingers in a circular or probing movement, all the areas of the big toe and particularly the upper and lower corners of the toe nail, relating respectively to the pineal and pituitary glands, and then massage down the spinal reflex and up the back of the heel to where the Achilles tendon is inserted into the heel bone. Massage will also be given from under the inner ankle bone over the top of the foot to below the outer ankle bone for the reflex to the pelvic girdle. Approximately 30 minutes will be spent massaging each foot in this manner. Massage will also be given to the head working up and down a line from the centre of the head to below the occipital ridge and along the base of the skull up the mastoid bones on each side. In addition, the hands may be worked on similarly to the feet — from the outer and inner corners of the thumb nail, down the outer edge of the thumb to the wrist and across the back of the wrist.

Using this method, the right foot is worked on first since it relates to the patterns which the person is working on in the present and what they are making of their life; the left foot relates to patterns not yet expressed which have been present since the person came into life.

Considerable publicity was achieved for this method of treatment for mentally-retarded children and although of benefit in this field it can also help people of all ages including women in pregnancy. Since it is not a complicated technique it can be used by families and friends but the possible effects from the massage should be understood.

Polarity Therapy

Polarity therapy was first described by the late Dr Randolph Stone in the 1940s and involves the stimulating and balancing of the body's life energy. It involves a complete system of health care using diet, exercise, manipulation and mental attitude. Dr Stone had studied Zone Therapy with Dr Fitzgerald and developed this work into a different system called Polarity Therapy which was so called since it involved the balancing of the electromagnetic currents of energy which flow backwards and forwards between the positive and negative poles of the body. The head is regarded as being positively charged and the feet as being negatively charged, so there is a tendency for energy to flow from head to feet. The feet become of great importance at the changeover points where energy flow is reversed. Dr Stone saw the ten longitudinal zones of Zone Therapy as bilateral energy channels created by the five chakras (energy centres). He also described nine horizontal zones in the body with the upper six horizontal zones being represented in the feet and hands as six horizontal zones. Each zone had a positive, negative or neutral charge and areas in the same horizontal zones of the same charge could be linked. This relationship is still considered significant for Reflexology by some schools of thought.

With polarity therapy, precise massage of reflex points is not involved but the two hands are placed on the body to redirect the energy flow. This pattern is also achieved in Reflexology treatment when one hand is used to apply pressure to a reflex point with the other hand on the other side of the foot supporting the area being worked on and in this way setting up a current of energy through the foot between the hands.

The interpretation of the direction for massage when giving Reflexology treatment in accordance with the principles of polarity therapy is probably not appropriate, though it is considered so by some schools of thought.

Massage

A general massage to the whole body as means of reducing tensions and causing relaxation will include massage to the feet and hands. The massage to these areas will not be as precise as for Reflexology massage when each reflex area will be worked on, but the general massage to the whole area of both feet and both hands will help to relax these areas and improve the flow of energy within these areas. Some therapists may, however, include the precise massage of Reflexology when giving general massage to the feet and hands.

The Vacuflex System

The Vacuflex System was developed by a Danish reflexologist, Inge Dougans, following six years of practising Reflexology. The system is seen not as a replacement for traditional Reflexology but as a complimentary method introducing modern techniques to the basic Reflexology principles. This system is sometimes known as the 'boot' treatment since it involves placing large felt boots on the feet which encase the whole foot and the ankle. Air is then removed from the boots by a vacuum pump creating equal pressure over the entire foot and thus massaging all the reflex areas in both feet with equal pressure. The treatment only takes about five minutes. On removal of the boots, markings and discolourations will be seen on the feet corresponding to the reflex zones which are out of balance and which would have been tender if massaged in the usual manner of Reflexology. These markings then offer a diagnosis of the imbalances present. The second stage of the treatment uses suction pads which are placed on the acupuncture meridian lines in the lower legs and arms to stimulate the body's vital energies. This second stage of the treatment takes about 20 minutes.

The system has similar results to Reflexology treatment and would perhaps appeal to a different group of people than standard Reflexology since it is of a shorter duration and involves equipment. Having experienced the relaxing benefits of an hour's massage of the feet with Reflexology treatment, the shorter mechanical approach might not appeal but certainly the effects can be considered as being comparable.

There will be other alternative therapies when the feet may be incorporated in the treatment procedure but the above are a few of the more likely therapies to include hand and foot work, though they should not be confused with true Reflexology treatment.

10 Reflexology Around the World

The popularity of Reflexology spreads world-wide and in most countries it is now possible to find a Reflexology practitioner. Many countries have an association or society for Reflexology practitioners. The laws governing the practice of alternative therapies do vary considerably in different parts of the world and in some countries the practitioner may be giving treatments when the laws of that country only allow medically trained people to offer forms of treatment. It does seem unfair that people can be penalized for doing good work which is of great benefit to others.

The following extracts taken from letters from Reflexology practitioners or students working in different countries describe briefly the degree of acceptance of Reflexology in their country.

In Switzerland, Reflexology is very popular and is taught in some of the nurses' training schools, as well as being taught to other groups. However, the laws governing the practice of Reflexology vary in each canton, with some allowing it and some not. In the cantons which do not allow Reflexology as a means of treatment, it is sometimes permitted as a means of relaxation provided that the term treatment or therapy is not mentioned.

In France, the regulations concerning the practice of alternative therapies are also very strict only allowing medically qualified persons to practice a method such as Reflexology.

In Italy, an active Reflexology association has become established, with Reflexology now well-known and popular, particularly in the large cities.

In Germany, training courses for Reflexology practitioners have been held for many years and an association exists. Natural therapies have always been popular in Germany with spa treatments and Reflexology is considered an acceptable form of massage treatment.

In Greece, there is a growing interest in Reflexology but as with other 'alternative' therapies, it is still in its infancy. It is possible to buy books and charts on the subject and people are interested in receiving treatment, though mainly those who have heard of the method in other countries. The orthodox medical practitioners do not, as yet, hold positive views about the benefits of treatment. Legally, Reflexology should not be practised by those not medically trained but the law is not always held to. Healthy eating has long been established in this country with an aversion to the introduction of unnatural, convenience foods, so the interest in natural therapies should become wider.

In Belgium, there is a great interest in Reflexology from people of all walks of life and the method is taught in some nursing schools. The people most interested in receiving treatment are those with a keen interest in alternative methods, those who have tried all other types of therapy without success, and in general more women are interested than men. The medical profession does not have a great regard for this type of treatment mainly as there is no scientific proof for it. Reflexology does not receive much media publicity but in the French part of Belgium there are three main centres where Reflexology is taught. The law only permits medical practitioners to practise alternative therapies but interest in these types of therapy is growing.

In Holland, alternative therapies are popular and accepted though no Reflexology association, as such, exists. There are a number of different training schools. The medical profession does not appear to have a very high regard for Reflexology but with the growing interest in the method, the good results which can be achieved may alter this view.

In Denmark, Reflexology is very popular and there are many practising Reflexologists. There are four main training schools including one which is only for nurses. In some hospitals, Reflexology treatment is incorporated into the treatment of patients. Of all the European countries, Denmark is probably the one where Reflexology is most widely accepted and well known and practitioners may work quite legally.

In South Africa, in recent years the method has become very popular with people from all backgrounds. There are three main training schools with associated societies and the legal practice of Reflexology varies in the different principalities. A licence to practise has to be issued to those wishing to set up a practice. The medical profession does not show strong opposition to alternative therapies though few regard them as having much value. The alternative practitioner is not legally allowed to diagnose. Some magazine publicity is given to Reflexology and most of those seeking treatment are those who have tried many other therapies for longstanding complaints but as the good results achieved are heard of others are also seeking treatment.

In Kenya, the interest in Reflexology is growing amongst all racial and cultural groups. Those training in the method are usually from medical or para-medical backgrounds and include nurses, masseurs, beauty therapists and some doctors. However, the medical profession do not formally recognize Reflexology as a therapy. In general, most practitioners would keep a low profile so as not to cause upset to the medical profession, which might lead to their practice being denounced.

In India, more and more people are becoming interested in Reflexology along with other natural therapies. The term Reflexology is not readily known but the method is usually represented by the term acupressure. The method is not criticized by medical practitioners and much publicity is now received for the method through the media and in particular newspapers. Natural medicine has always been known in India so the acceptance of therapies such as Reflexology is not difficult. There is no actual Reflexology association in India but the method is taught alongside other similar therapies.

In America, as with all 'alternative' therapies, there is much interest in Reflexology treatment. There are many training schools and therapists have to have a licence to practise in most states.

Reflexology is also practised in many other countries including Australia, New Zealand, Canada, Brazil, Uruguay, Japan, Israel, Austria and Sweden. It is uncertain, however, as to whether or not Reflexology in its present form is practised in China. Although based on a system of oriental medicine, the method does not appear to be used as a system on its own but is probably incorporated into other methods used.

It is therefore clear that Reflexology is known to people in many parts of the world and as word spreads of the successes which it can achieve, more and more people are seeking treatment. It is disappointing that some countries do not allow the practice of the method since in the hands of a trained practitioner this simple massage method can have amazing results. It must surely become accepted that any method which is going to help the health of a person should be considered and that whether the method is allopathic (traditional western medicine) or an 'alternative' therapy, the practitioner is working for the good of the person and to achieve good health, and to maintain good health must be a wish of nearly everyone. The 'alternative' therapies such as Reflexology have much to offer to people keen to care for themselves in a natural manner.

Useful Addresses

For further information on Reflexology practitioners and training courses, the following addresses may be of help:

The Bayly School of Reflexology,
Monks Orchard,
Whitbourne,
Worcester WR6 5RB

The Bayly School is the official teaching body of the British Reflexology Association and a register of members of the Association, published yearly (price £1.00), can be obtained from the School. This Association also has an overseas membership. Other associations, training schools and practitioners with which the Bayly School has contact but not necessarily a direct link are:

L'ASER (L'Association Suisse pour l'Etude de la Reflexologie),
President: Noelle Weyeneth,
214 route des convers,
2616 Renan,
Switzerland.

CIRF (Centro Italiano Riflessologia Fitzgerald),
Director: Erasmo Buzzacchi,
via Bronzino 11,
20133 Milan,
Italy.

South African Reflexology Society,
  Mrs Inge Dougans,
  Shop 4, Medical Centre Ext,
  50 Kings Road,
  Pinetown 3600,
  Republic of South Africa.

Mrs Catherine Wade,
  P.O. Box 15020,
  Nairobi, Kenya.

Index

acne 37, 124
acupressure/acupuncture 167-71
adrenal gland 76-9
allergies 37, 79, 124, 125, 156, 157
angina 124, 125
anorexia 124, 125
appendix 70, 71
arm 44-6, 82
aromatherapy 167, 171, 172
arthritis 49, 79, 85, 123, 125
asthma 53, 124, 126, 157

backache 123, 126, 157, 158
Bayly, Doreen 18
Bell's palsy 123, 127
bladder 72, 73
brain 30, 31
breast 92, 95, 96
breast cysts 124, 127
bronchi 52, 53
bronchitis 53, 124, 127
bursitis 123, 127

cancer 124, 128
cataract 40
catarrh 37, 70, 123, 128
chilblains 124, 128, 158
colitis 124, 128

coma 123, 129
conjunctivitis 40, 123, 129
constipation 70, 72, 124, 129,
  158, 159
cough 124, 129
cramp 123, 130
crystal deposits 115
cystitis 124, 130, 159

deafness 33, 41, 123, 130
depression 97, 123, 130, 159, 160
dermatitis 124, 131
diabetes 65, 124, 131
diagnosis 116
diaphragm 54, 55
diarrhoea 72, 124, 131
diverticulitis 132

ears 40, 41
earache 41, 123, 132
eczema 97, 124, 132
elbow 45, 46
emphysema 53, 124, 132
epilepsy 123, 133
Eustachian tube 40, 41
eyes 37-40
eye strain 123, 133

face 36, 37
Fallopian tube 92, 95
fibroids 89, 124, 133
fibrositis 123, 133
Fitzgerald, Dr William 12, 13, 15
flatulence 124, 134
foot,
   bones of 22, 23, 113, 114
   chart of reflex areas 99-100
   problems 112, 123, 134
fractures 123, 134

gall bladder 61, 62
gall stones 124, 135
glaucoma 40, 123, 135
goitre 46, 124, 135
gout 123, 136

haemorrhoids 124, 137
hand,
   bones of 25, 26
   chart of reflex areas 101-2
hay fever 37, 123, 136, 160, 161
head 30, 31
headaches 32, 37, 123, 136
heart 56-8
heart attack 58, 124, 136
hepatitis 61, 124, 137
hernia 124, 137
hip 83-6
history of method 11, 12
hypertension 58, 124, 138
hypoglycaemia 65, 124, 138
hypotension 58, 124, 139

ileo-caecal valve 70, 71
incontinence 73, 124, 139

indigestion 66, 124, 139
infection 62, 124, 140
infertility 87, 95, 124, 140
Ingham, Eunice 12, 18, 20
insomnia 30, 123, 140, 161
intestine,
   large 70-2
   small 66, 67, 70

jaundice 61, 124, 141

kidney 75, 76
kidney stones 49, 75, 124, 140
Kirlian photography 118, 119
knee 84, 85
knee pains 123, 140, 161

liver 59-61
lumbago 123, 141
lung 49, 52, 53
lymphatic system 92, 93, 96, 97

Marquardt, Hanne 20
massage 167, 174
mastitis 124, 142
Ménière's disease 123, 142
meningitis 123, 142
menopause 87, 89, 124, 142
menstrual problems 87, 89, 124,
   143
metamorphic technique 167, 172,
   173
migraine 32, 123, 143, 161
multiple sclerosis 123, 144
muscle strains 123, 144

neck 31, 32

neck stiffness 123, 144, 161
nephritis 124, 145
neuralgia 37, 123, 145

oesophagus 51, 66
ovary 86, 87
ovarian cysts 87, 124, 145

pancreas 62-5
paralysis 123, 145
parathyroid gland 48, 49
Parkinson's disease 32, 123, 146
pelvic region, muscles of 83, 84
phlebitis 124, 146
pituitary gland 29, 30
pleurisy 53, 124, 146
polarity therapy 167, 173, 174
pregnancy 89, 124, 147
pre-menstrual tension 124, 147, 163
preventative therapy 116-17
prostate gland 89, 90, 91
  enlargement of 91, 124, 147
psoriasis 97, 124, 148

Raynaud's disease 124, 148
rectum 72
rheumatism 49, 123, 148
rhinitis 123, 149
ribs 53, 54

sacro-iliac joint 82, 83
sciatic nerve 78, 79, 83, 85
sciatica 79, 85, 123, 149, 163
shiatsu 167-71
shingles 124, 150
shoulder 43, 44, 81
  frozen 123, 134, 160

sinuses 37, 38
sinusitis 37, 70, 123, 150, 164
skin 97
solar plexus 55, 56
spine 33-5, 88
spleen 62, 63
spondylitis 123, 150
sternum 53, 54
stomach 65, 66
stroke 32, 123, 151

tear duct, blocked 40, 123, 151, 164
teeth 42, 43
tennis elbow 46, 123, 152
tenosynovitis 123, 151
tension 115, 124, 152
testes 87, 88
thrombosis 124, 152
thymus gland 58, 59
thyroid gland 46, 47
  imbalances of 46, 124, 153,
    164, 165
tinnitus 41, 123, 153, 165-6
tonsilitis 124, 154, 165
toothache 37, 43, 123, 154
trachea 49, 52
treatment,
  length of 120-21
  order of 27, 28, 97-8
  position for 120
  reactions to 117-18
  self 122
  sensations of 103-9
  techniques for 110-11

ulcers 66, 124, 154
ureter tube 74, 75

uterus 88, 89, 91

vacuflex system 167, 175
varicose veins 124, 155
vertigo 41, 123, 155, 166

zones,
   longitudinal 13-16, 115
   transverse 20-4, 29, 49, 66
zone related areas 18, 19
zone therapy 12, 13, 15, 17, 18

Sharon Faelton
The Allergy Self-Help Book   £4.99

A STEP-BY-STEP GUIDE TO DRUG-FREE RELIEF OF
ASTHMA, HAY FEVER, HEADACHES, FATIGUE, DIGESTIVE
DISORDERS AND OVER 50 OTHER ALLERGY-RELATED
HEALTH PROBLEMS

Self-help can do more for allergies than for any other form of
disease. The more you learn about the cause of your trouble — and
exactly how to avoid whatever irritates you — the less likely you
are to need constant medical supervision.

This comprehensive, easy-to-use guide — based on firsthand
interviews with and reports from some of the world's most
experienced allergy doctors — will help you identify the specific
food or environmental substance that's the cause of your discomfort
or your child's — and tell you what you can do about it. It includes
a special no-allergy diet plan and expert advice on how to decode
lists of ingredients on food labels to avoid hidden food allergens,
how to manage food allergies in children, and how to choose safe
household cleaning products and cosmetics.

There are plenty of helpful, practical tips on how to escape harmful
airborne particles, some of which you may not even know exist,
and the book ends with a unique A-Z of allergic reactions that can
mimic any of over 50 different health complaints, including
arthritis, depression, eczema, insomnia, migraine, sinusitis and
vertigo.

Peter G. Hanson M.D.
The Joy of Stress £3.99

*How to use stress to generate energy and achieve greater health,
wealth and happiness.*
*Use the Hanson method to add more years to your life and more
life to your years . . .*

The mismanagement of stress can be fatal. Under stress, people
don't feel at their peak, they don't perform at work to the best of
their abilities, they are more likely to be sick, and ultimately they
are most likely to die before their time.

But you can make the stresses in your life work positively for you.
Dr Hanson's easy-to-read and entertaining book shows you how to
harness stress productively. It distils scientific facts into practical
advice for everyone — making sense out of the confusing and often
contradictory advice we've all been subjected to on stress, body
management, longevity, productivity, and nutrition.

The key to surviving and thriving on stress is control. The Hanson
Method teaches you how to ignore what you can't control, and to
control what you can. It's a *practical* plan that you can put to work
immediately and continue to use forever. So don't hide from
stresses; go out and challenge new ones. Take the *thrill* from stress,
but leave the *threat* behind. Thrive under pressure and learn the
true Joy of Stress!

FIRST BRITISH PUBLICATION

D.C. Jarvis M.D.
Folk Medicine   £2.50

The honey and cider-vinegar way to health.
Over half-a-million copies sold!
Health secrets which can prolong life and give vigour to young and
old . . .

The late Dr Jarvis lived and practised among the tough mountain
folk of Vermont for over fifty years. This unique and remarkable
book — which has sold over 500,000 copies in the Pan edition
alone — is the result of his deep study of their way of life, and in
particular of their concept of diet and time-honoured folk medicine.

It offers a novel theory on the treatment and prevention of a wide
range of diseases and nagging complaints —

THE COMMON COLD
HAY FEVER
ARTHRITIS
KIDNEY TROUBLE
DIGESTIVE DISORDERS
OVERWEIGHT
HIGH BLOOD PRESSURE
CHRONIC FATIGUE

and many others which often defy conventional diagnosis and
treatment.

'There is not a family in the land who won't find its theories —
and propositions — fascinating' DAILY EXPRESS

Valerie Ann Worwood
Aromantics   £4.95

Add zest, romance and fun to your life with nature's quintessential oils

Quintessential oils are pure substances distilled from plants, and they have been used throughout history. They offer natural cures to ailments that many of us commonly suffer – and they smell divine.

But quintessential oils have other properties – they're not used for medicinal reasons alone. Do you need to put more zest into your day, or to enrich a romantic evening? *Aromantics* explains how aromatic oils can relax, tone and invigorate your whole body, how to choose oils to suit you and your lover, how perfumes, oils and massage can enhance your lovemaking and bring relief from tiredness and stress. In this book you will find hundreds of oils and blends to use for health and happiness. There are even suggestions for aromatic aphrodisiac food and wines that you can make, and there is full information on how and where to obtain the best quintessential oils.

Aromantics is about nature and romance, and attracting a particular sexual partner using these oils. It's relaxation and excitation, creating a harmony of body and mind, sensuality and, yes, sex. So bring out your true Aromantic self – vital, happy, and in control of life and love!

Oliver Sacks
Migraine: Understanding the Common Disorder £3.95

A Practical Guide to Treatment and Relief
        'Balanced, authoritative . . . brilliant' THE TIMES

'Written by one of the great clinical writers of the 20th century,
Migraine, intended for the general public, should be read as much
for its brilliant insights into the nature of our mental functioning as
for its discussion of migraine' NEW YORK TIMES BOOK
REVIEW

A new revised edition of Oliver Sacks' classic book on migraine,
this is a full and penetrating insight into that most distressing of
common illnesses. The symptoms, treatments and psychological
effects are all discussed in detail, making it an essential guide to the
migraine sufferer who wants to know exactly what he or she is up
against.

'Informative, well-written and entertaining — includes a good
review of specific drug treatments and can be read by all those who
have to deal with migraine' THE LANCET

'A most excellent survey . . . must be the definitive book on the
subject' NURSING MIRROR

'Well organised, original, constructive . . . deserves a wide
readership' MENTAL HEALTH

'His commentary is so erudite, so gracefully written, that even
those people fortunate enough to never have had a migraine in their
lives should find it equally compelling' NEW YORK TIMES

All Pan books are available at your local bookshop or newsagent, or can be ordered direct from the publisher. Indicate the number of copies required and fill in the form below:

Send to: **CS Department, Pan Books Ltd., P.O. Box 40, Basingstoke, Hants.   RG21 2YT.**

or phone: 0256 469551 (Ansaphone), quoting title, author and Credit Card number.

Please enclose a remittance* to the value of the cover price plus: 60p for the first book plus 30p per copy for each additional book ordered to a maximum charge of £2.40 to cover postage and packing.

*Payment may be made in sterling by UK personal cheque, postal order, sterling draft or international money order, made payable to Pan Books Ltd.

Alternatively by Barclaycard/Access:

Card No. | | | | | | | | | | | | | | | | | | |

Signature:

Applicable only in the UK and Republic of Ireland.

While every effort is made to keep prices low, it is sometimes necessary to increase prices at short notice. Pan Books reserve the right to show on covers and charge new retail prices which may differ from those advertised in the text or elsewhere.

NAME AND ADDRESS IN BLOCK LETTERS PLEASE:

....

Name ———————————————————————————————

Address ———————————————————————————————

———————————————————————————————

———————————————————————————————

———————————————————————————————

3/87